Echocardiography

Review

APPLETON DAVIES INC.

Echocardiography
Review

Barton A. Bean, RVT

Past President, Society of Non-Invasive Vascular Technology
President, Answers Company
Director, BBI Vascular Laboratory
Anaheim, California
Editor

Kathleen A. Oss, BS, RDMS

Medical Education Consultant
K. Oss and Associates
Seattle, Washington
Associate Editor

Appleton Davies, Inc.
Publishers in Medicine and Surgery
Pasadena, California

Library of Congress Cataloging-in-Publication Data

Echocardiography review.

Includes bibliographical references.
1. Echocardiography—Examinations, questions, etc.
I. Bean, Barton A. II. Oss, Kathleen A., 1950-
[DNLM: 1. Echocardiography—examination questions. WG 18 E18]
RC683.5.U5E244   1989   616.1'207543'076   89-18089
ISBN 0-941022-16-1

Appleton Davies, Inc.
Publishers in Medicine and Surgery
32 South Raymond Avenue
Pasadena, California 91105

Copy editing by Lillian R. Rodberg & Associates.

Printed and bound in the United States of America.

ISBN 0-941022-16-1

CONTRIBUTORS

Barton A. Bean, RVT
Past President, Society of Non-Invasive
    Vascular Technology
President, Answers Company
Director, BBI Vascular Laboratory
Anaheim, California

Sandra Baker
Echocardiographer
Ultrasound Consultants
Huntington Beach, California

John B. Bennett, III, PhD
Cardiovascular Physiologist
South Norwalk, Connecticut

Sandra Hagen-Ansert, BA, RDMS
Pediatric Echocardiography
University of California Medical Center
San Diego, California

Thomas Lonergan, BS
Director, Department of Cardiology
Downey Community Hospital
Downey, California

Carol Mortier, BS, RDMS
Cardiovascular Group of Southern
    California
Beverly Hills, California

Kathleen A. Oss, BS, RDMS
Medical Education Consultant
K. Oss and Associates
Seattle, Washington

David Sahn, MD
Chief, Division of Pediatric Cardiology
University of California Medical Center
San Diego, California

PREFACE

With questions, answers, brief explanations, and references presented in the form of an examination, *Echocardiography Review* is designed to assess the state of one's professional knowledge and to provide direction for further study. Specifically, we wrote this self-assessment review to help registry candidates prepare for their certification examination. But students, registered echocardiographers, ultrasonographers, and others in the medical community might well find this review to be a valuable means of learning more about echocardiography and of keeping current with this evolving discipline.

How To Use This Book

The review is organized into two main parts, *Echocardiography* and *The Physics of Ultrasound*, with 20 chapters on key topics. Part III, which is printed on colored paper for easy reference, contains the answers to the questions in the first two parts, as well as explanations and references.

Whether you are using this book to prepare for your registry examination or to keep current, the best strategy is to pretend that the book *is* an examination: Answer all of the questions in one sitting and then—and only then—score the answers to identify your strengths and weaknesses. (Avoid the temptation to browse among questions and answers, for that will only undermine the value of the book and dissipate your energies.) Then, referring to the suggested sources for further study, design an efficient and realistic program of study to update your knowledge and to ensure an informed and confident performance on the registry examination.

We have designed this book and the exercise that it represents to help build conceptual understanding, not to coach candidates in memorizing answers to specific questions. No one who uses this book should assume that the questions herein will appear on the registry examination or that the act of learning the answers by rote will assure the candidate of a passing score. Rather, we hope that you will use *Echocardiography Review* to strengthen your understanding of the concepts, principles, and practice of echocardiography. Although it is important to commit certain facts, figures, and formulas to memory, that task is immeasurably easier when one has a strong conceptual understanding of the subject.

Types of Questions

Both the registry examination and this review contain three types of questions: A-type (conventional multiple-choice questions), X-type (a series of true/false questions based on one preceding statement), and true/false questions that are not in the X-type format.

A-type questions consist of a *stem* (which appears in boldface type in the examples below) and several possible answers, only one of which is correct unless the stem says otherwise. Example:

1. **The American Society of Echocardiography adopted the "leading edge" method of measurement because:**

   A. People were turning up the gain too much.
   B. The nature of the interaction between ultrasound and anatomic interfaces makes it the best method.
   C. The advent of gray-scale M mode made it possible.
   D. It produces the most consistent and reproducible measurements.

X-type questions, on the other hand, require you to answer *true* or *false* for each numbered question that follows the stem, as here:

Tricuspid valve echo findings in patients with such acquired diseases as endomyocardial fibrosis, endocardial fibroelastosis, and malignant carcinoid include: (True or False)

1. Increased E to A ratio.
2. Thickened leaflets and chordae.
3. Diastolic leaflet doming.
4. Restriction of leaflet motion.

Each time you see a numbered statement following the stem of an X-type question, remember to answer with *true* or *false*.

Finally, there are true/false questions that appear as single statements rather than in the X-type format. Example:

1. **Early diastolic murmurs are the result of aortic or pulmonary insufficiency.**
   True or False

In this case you would answer *true* or *false* and then proceed to the next question.

Strategies for Answering Questions

Whether you are studying for or actually taking a test, you should first try to provide the answer for the stem *without* looking at the choices provided. Doing this will help you recognize the appropriate answer.

The second strategy for successful test-taking is to answer all of the questions in a section for which the answer comes easily to you. Go through the *entire section* you are working on and answer as quickly as you can. Skip the questions about which you have doubts. By using this strategy you will be sure to leave no blanks for answers you *do* know, and your answers may trigger information that will help you when you go back to the questions that caused you more difficulty.

Next, go back and again answer the easiest of the remaining questions. Do this once or twice before tackling questions about which you are in a complete fog. Only then call on the science of probability to work in your behalf:

1. For each question, eliminate those answers you are sure are impossible.

2. Maybe that will leave only one answer, but if it leaves more than one: GUESS! (That is, you guess if you are actually taking the test; if you are studying, consult the answers, explanations, and references.)

Statistically, your first answer is most often correct, so do not change an answer unless you are absolutely certain you know what is correct.

Strategies for Taking Multiple-Choice Examinations

With any multiple-choice examination, certain psychological and practical strategies can enhance your performance. Follow these summarized rules to guarantee yourself the best possible test score:

1. Have enough pencils!
2. Eat lightly before the test so that you do not fall asleep.
3. Read all directions *very* carefully.
4. Try to answer the stem without looking at the answer choices; then try for the closest match.
5. Go through the entire section available to you, answering all of the easy questions.
6. Do step 5 again. Then again.
7. Return to the difficult questions and eliminate the answers you know are inappropriate.
8. When in doubt, finally, *guess.*
9. Ten minutes before the end of the test, answer *all* questions.
10. Do *not* go back to second-guess yourself. You will be wrong most of the time when you do this.

This book required the dedicated efforts of a group of seven expert contributors who worked hard and long to provide challenging, thought-provoking questions and clear, informative answers. It is with gratitude that I acknowledge them here. In particular, I thank my associate editor Kathy Oss, RDMS, without whose help this book would not have been completed.

Good skill!

Barton A. Bean, RVT

TABLE OF CONTENTS

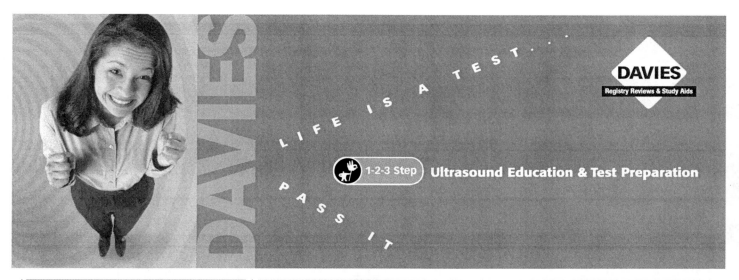

RVT

Vascular Technology

An Illustrated Review

Claudia Rumwell, RN, RVT
Michalene McPharlin, RN, RVT

Exam: Vascular Technology
Purpose: Single-source text
CME Credit: 12 hours

Here's the new 3rd Edition of the only concise textbook-style review based on the ARDMS outline of exam content. This new edition reviews and illustrates what you need to know to pass the Vascular Technology exam topic by topic, in one volume, by leading technologists who themselves have taken, passed, and helped others prepare for and pass their RVT exams. Includes case examples and self-assessment quizzes. Particularly useful in combination with *Vascular Technology Review*, *Vascular Physics Review*, and *ScoreCards*. 322 pp, **$69.95.**

ScoreCards™
for Vascular Technology

Cindy Owen, RDMS, RVT
D. E. Strandness, Jr., MD

CME Credit: 7.5 hours

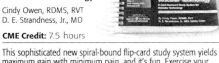

This sophisticated new spiral-bound flip-card study system yields maximum gain with minimum pain, and it's fun. Exercise your ability to think fast, recall key facts, and apply knowledge wherever you are. Highly portable, *ScoreCards* delivers more than 400 Q&A items keyed to the new registry outline, 50 image-based questions in the *Image Gallery*, explanations, and references. 854 pp, **$49.95.**

Vascular Technology Review

Don Ridgway, RVT
D. E. Strandness, Jr., MD

Exam: Vascular Technology
Purpose: Mock exam
CME Credit: 12 hours

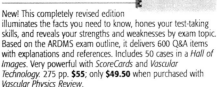

New! This completely revised edition illuminates the facts you need to know, hones your test-taking skills, and reveals your strengths and weaknesses by exam topic. Based on the ARDMS exam outline, it delivers 600 Q&A items with explanations and references. Includes 50 cases in a *Hall of Images*. Very powerful with *ScoreCards* and *Vascular Technology*. 275 pp. **$55;** only **$49.50** when purchased with *Vascular Physics Review*.

Vascular Physics Review

edited by Barton A. Bean, RVT

Exam: Vascular Physics
Purpose: Mock exam
CME Credit: 7.5 hours

Here's the vascular physics review candidates rely on. Approximately 500 illustrated question/answer/explanation items in registry format to simulate the exam so you can test yourself before taking the vascular physics exam. 180 pp. **$55;** **$49.50** when purchased with *Vascular Technology Review*.

RDMS

Ultrasound Physics Review

Cindy Owen, RVT, RDMS
James A. Zagzebski, PhD

Exam: Ultrasound Physics
Purpose: Mock exam
CME Credit: 12 hours

Looking for guidance and a clear understanding of this difficult topic? With registry-like questions, 100+ images, and simple explanations, *Ultrasound Physics Review* explains the facts you need to know to pass the registry exam from the sonographer's point of view. Precisely based on the ARDMS exam outline, *UPR* assesses your strengths and weaknesses by exam topic, hones your test-taking skills, and measures your progress. You won't be disappointed. 550 Q&A items with references. **$55;** only **$49.50** when purchased with another mock exam or any Fear of Physics text.

Abdominal Sonography Review

Cindy Owen, RVT, RDMS
Edward G. Grant, MD

Exam: Abdomen
Purpose: Mock exam
CME Credit: 12 hours

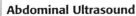

Strongly recommended! Based on the ARDMS abdomen specialty exam outline, this new edition contains 550 questions in registry format together with answers, thorough explanations, and quick references for further study. More than 60 image-based cases prepare you to tackle the images on the exam. Especially effective in combination with *Ultrasound Physics Review.* **$55;** only **$49.50** when purchased with *Ultrasound Physics Review.*

Ob/Gyn Sonography Review

Gill/Sliman/Callen

Exam: Ob/Gyn
Purpose: Mock exam
CME Credit: 12 hours

New! This registry-like practice exam by Gill, Callen and Sliman hones your test-taking skills and illuminates the facts and principles you must know to pass the ob/gyn specialty exam. Precisely based on the ARDMS exam outline, it focuses your efforts on what really counts. More than 515 questions in registry format with clear explanations and references. 100 image-based questions prepare you for the scans on your exam. 12 hours SDMS-approved CME. **$55** alone; **$49.50** when purchased with *Ultrasound Physics Review* or *Abdominal Sonography Review.*

RDMS, RDCS, RVT

Ob/Gyn Sonography

An Illustrated Review

Marie De Lange, BS, RDMS, RDCS
Glenn A. Rouse, MD

Exam: Ob/Gyn
Purpose: Single-source text
CME Credit: 12 hours

Just published! This new book serves several purposes with style and economy. It's a topic-by-topic review for the ARDMS exam, a concise text for training and cross-training, a clinical reference for practicing sonographers, a resource for interpreting physicians, and a convenient and inexpensive way to earn 12 hours' CME credit. First and foremost, it's a powerful registry-prep text. 384 pp. **$69.95.**

Abdominal Ultrasound

A Practitioner's Guide

Kathryn Gill, MS, RT, RDMS

Exam: Abdomen
Purpose: Textbook
CME Credit: 16 hours

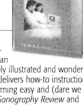

A great new book in full color with something for everyone—exam candidates, sonographers in training, veteran sonographers, and educators. Superbly illustrated and wonderfully written, *Abdominal Ultrasound* delivers how-to instruction and dozens of features that make learning easy and (dare we say it?) fun. Perfect with *Abdominal Sonography Review* and *Ultrasound Physics Review*, it covers all exam topics. 1,000+ illustrations. Saunders. 474 pp, **$102.**

Echocardiography Review

Barton A. Bean, RVT
Kathleen Oss, BS, RDMS

Exam: Adult Echo
Purpose: Mock exam

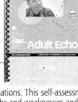

An indispensable resource for RDCS candidates containing 679 questions, answers, and brief explanations. This self-assessment study manual identifies your strengths and weaknesses and lets you test yourself before you take the registry exam. Especially useful with *Ultrasound Physics Review*. **$55;** only **$49.50** when purchased with any other mock exam.

Fear of Physics?

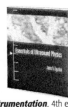

Combine *Ultrasound Physics Review.* with one of the three best physics textbooks available: >*Essentials of Ultrasound Physics*, by James A. Zagzebski, PhD. A short, simple, clear, and well-illustrated intro. Perfect for physicsphobes. Mosby. 234 pp, **$51.95.** >*Ultrasound Physics & Instrumentation*, 4th ed., by Wayne R. Hedrick, PhD, et al. Well written and easy to understand, but broader and more complex than Zagzebski. For middle-of-the-roaders. Mosby. 445 pp, **$62.95.** >*Diagnostic Ultrasound: Principles & Instruments*, by Frederick Kremkau, PhD. Thorough, comprehensive, classic—the standard and "most trusted" physics text, now in a new edition. For the serious student. Saunders. 442 pp, **$59.95.**

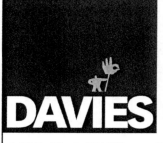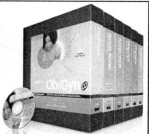

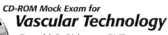
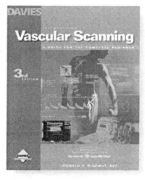

PART I

ECHOCARDIOGRAPHY

ONE

ANATOMY, PHYSIOLOGY, AND CLINICAL INDICATIONS

1.0 The American Society of Echocardiography adopted the "leading edge" method of measurement because:

    A. People were turning up the gain too much.
    B. The nature of the interaction between ultrasound and anatomical interfaces makes this advisable.
    C. The advent of gray scale M mode made this possible.
    D. It produces the most consistent and reproducible measurements.

1.1 The term *basilar area of the ventricle* refers to the:

    A. Ventricular myocardium at the apex.
    B. Mid segments of the ventricle.
    C. Ventricular myocardium at the atrioventricular valves.
    D. None of the above.

1.2 The infundibulum is related to the area of the right ventricle called the:

    A. Inflow tract.
    B. Outflow tract.
    C. Apical area.
    D. Subvalvular area.

1.3 The three primary branches of the aortic arch include all of the following EXCEPT the:

    A. Innominate artery.
    B. Right subclavian artery.
    C. Left common carotid artery.
    D. Left subclavian artery.

1.4 The term *tunica adventitia* refers to:

    A. The inner lining of the arterial wall.
    B. The outer lining of the arterial wall.
    C. Transverse arterial muscle fibers.
    D. The intimal wall.
    E. The middle layer of the arterial wall.

1.5 The term *tunica intima* refers to which of the following:

    A. The inner lining of the arterial wall.
    B. The outer lining of the arterial wall.
    C. Transverse arterial muscle fibers.
    D. Longitudinal muscle fibers.
    E. The middle layer of the arterial wall.

1.6 Dextracardia indicates:

    A. Enlargement of all cardiac chambers.
    B. An abnormal conduction system.
    C. Heart located in the right side of the chest.
    D. Dual chambers of the right ventricle.

1.7 You are asked to pay particular attention to the semilunar valves. These valves are the:

    A. Mitral and aortic valves.
    B. Mitral and tricuspid valves.
    C. Pulmonic and tricuspid valves.
    D. Aortic and pulmonic valves.

1.8 The great vessels of the heart are the:

        A. Inferior vena cava and superior vena cava.
        B. Inferior vena cava and subclavian artery.
        C. Aorta and subclavian artery.
        D. Aorta and pulmonary artery.

1.9 Name and label each point on the anterior mitral valve leaflet:

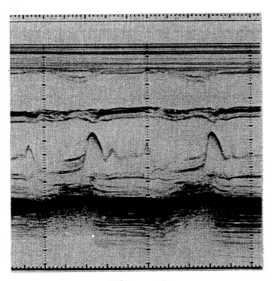

Figure 1

1.10 Name and label the three walls transected by the transducer at midventricular level:

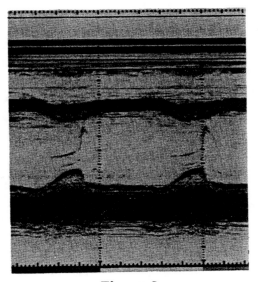

Figure 2

1.11 Name and label all structures and chambers transected by the M-mode ultrasound beam directed through the base of the heart:

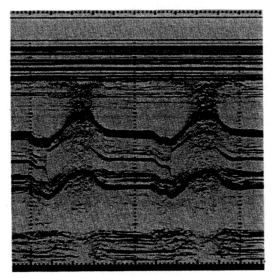

Figure 3

1.12 In M mode, the structure used to pinpoint end systole for measurement is:

    A. The R wave of the ECG.
    B. Maximum anterior motion of the left ventricular posterior wall.
    C. Maximum posterior motion of the interventricular septum.
    D. The Q wave of the ECG.

1.13 The motion of the septum should be evaluated by M mode at the:

    A. Basal level.
    B. Mitral level.
    C. Midventricular level.
    D. Apical level.

1.14 The coronary sinus returns blood to the left atrium.

    True or False

1.15 The ostium of the coronary arteries may sometimes be visualized in a short-axis two-dimensional echo view at the level of the aortic valve.

True or False

1.16 Since phases of the cardiac cycle are discussed in terms of systole and diastole of the ventricle, what phase would be occurring during atrial filling?

A. Diastole.
B. Systole.
C. Insovolumic phase.

1.17 In the ECG cycle, late ventricular filling occurs after the:

A. P wave.
B. Q wave.
C. R wave.
D. T wave.

If a patient presents with an early diastolic murmur you would concentrate interest on the: (True or False)

1.18 Aortic valve.
1.19 Mitral valve.
1.20 Tricuspid valve.
1.21 Pulmonic valve.

1.22 Which valve would you suspect to be abnormal if auscultation revealed an Austin-Flint murmur?

A. Aortic valve.
B. Mitral valve.
C. Tricuspid valve.
D. Pulmonic valve.

1.23 Most authors consider the major components of the first heart sound to be:

    A. Closure of the semilunar valves.
    B. Closure of the atrioventricular valves.
    C. Opening of the semilunar valves.
    D. Opening of the atrioventricular valves.

1.24 The heart sound most often associated with mitral valve prolapse is:

    A. Gallop rhythm.
    B. Ejection sounds.
    C. Opening snap.
    D. Systolic click.

1.25 The heart sound associated with mitral and/or tricuspid stenosis is:

    A. Ejection sound.
    B. Gallop rhythm.
    C. A friction rub.
    D. Opening snap.

1.26 Early diastolic murmurs are due to aortic or pulmonic insufficiency.

    True or False

Myxomas are the most common type of cardiac tumor. They comprise half of all reported cases. Which of the following statements are true? (True or False)

    1.27 These tumors can be located either inside or outside the heart.
    1.28 Approximately 40% of patients with left atrial myxomas have systemic emboli to the brain or extremities.
    1.29 Myxomas occur only in the left atrium.
    1.30 Females are affected slightly more often than males.

Symptoms associated with pericarditis include: (True or False)

1.31 A severe, sharp pain located precordially that may radiate into the shoulders and neck.

1.32 Ankle swelling.

1.33 Changing positions and taking deep breaths increases the pain.

1.34 The pain is dull and radiates into the jaw.

Symptoms noted with mitral valve prolapse syndrome include: (True or False)

1.35 Palpitations and sharp pain unrelated to exercise.

1.36 Lower back pain and headache.

1.37 Fatigue and dyspnea.

1.38 Palpitations and dizzy spells.

1.39 A pseudonym for mitral valve prolapse syndrome is:

    A. Ebstein's anomaly.
    B. Barlow's syndrome.
    C. Crohn's disease.
    D. Prinzmetal angina.

1.40 The term *trepopnea* is the sensation of dyspnea or palpitation, or an uncomfortable feeling that may occur when patients with cardiac diseases lie on their left side.

    True or False

1.41 The term *dyspnea* refers to the condition of:

    A. Difficulty in digesting food.
    B. Difficulty in breathing.
    C. Rapid breathing.
    D. Deep breathing.

1.42 If a patient awakens in the night with shortness of breath, 1 to 2 hours after falling asleep, what disease might be suspected?

    A. Angina pectoris.
    B. Mitral valve prolapse.
    C. Constrictive pericarditis.
    D. Congestive heart failure.

1.43 Anemia or cyanosis may be a manifestation of serious underlying heart disease.

    True or False

Palpation of arterial pulses is a method used to help determine the presence or absence of diagnostic physical signs for certain cardiac diseases. Which of the following statements is/are correct? (True or False)

    1.44 Heart failure, obstruction of flow by valvular stenosis, and constrictive pericarditis can cause a diminished stroke volume.
    1.45 Normal peripheral pulses arrive later than the carotid pulse.
    1.46 Pulsus alternans implies impaired ventricular function and is often present in massive pericardial effusion, particularly pericardial tamponade.
    1.47 Aortic regurgitation and carotid atherosclerosis cause a large stroke volume, wide pulse pressure, and lowered peripheral resistance with resultant bounding hyperkinetic pulses.

1.48 Dextrocardia can be detected by chest x-ray, percussion, ECG examination, auscultation, and asking the patient.

    True or False

Which of the following signs are indicative but not diagnostic of heart disease? (True or False)

    1.49 Sharp chest pains.
    1.50 Cyanosis.
    1.51 Clubbing.
    1.52 Obesity.

1.53 Which one of the following is most likely to cause a decrease in cardiac output?

    A. A decrease in peripheral resistance.
    B. Hyperemia.
    C. Decrease in left ventricular stroke volume.
    D. Increase in heart rate.
    E. Hypertension.

1.54 A decrease in left ventricular contractility secondary to acute myocardial infarction will:

    A. Increase cardiac output (Q) by increasing resistance (R).
    B. Decrease cardiac output (Q) by decreasing pressure (delta P).
    C. Increase velocity of flow in the aorta.
    D. Decrease delta P with no effect on cardiac output (Q).

1.55 If all other factors remain constant, you would expect a reduction in vessel diameter to:

    A. Increase velocity.
    B. Decrease the likelihood of turbulence.
    C. Decrease viscosity.
    D. Decrease kinetic energy.
    E. Increase flow.

1.56 Which one of the following is most likely to cause turbulent flow of blood in the aorta ?

    A. An increase in cardiac output from 5 L/min to 20 L/min.
    B. An increase in hematocrit.
    C. A decrease in cardiac output to one-half of normal.
    D. An increase in arterial pressure of 5 mm Hg.
    E. A hypertensive episode.

Which of the following are characteristics of turbulent flow? (True or False)

    1.57 It can be predicted by Reynold's number.
    1.58 It is responsible for murmurs, bruits and thrills.
    1.59 It increases pressure downstream.
    1.60 It occurs where there are abrupt variations in vessel diameter.
    1.61 It is affected by velocity.

1.62 During an experiment, a laboratory animal suddenly develops 2:1 heart block, effectively reducing heart rate by one-half. Which ONE of the following responses would account for pressure being maintained at the same level as before the heart block?

    A. Peripheral resistance decreased by one-half.
    B. Massive vasodilatation of the arterial sphincters.
    C. Peripheral resistance doubled.
    D. Arteriovenous shunting.
    E. Peripheral resistance unchanged.

1.63 A subject has a cardiac output of 5 L/min at a heart rate of 75 beats/min. If stroke volume remains constant, what will be the effect of an increase in heart rate to 150 beats per minute?

    A. Cardiac output would increase to 22.5 L/min.
    B. Cardiac output would increase to 25 L/min.
    C. Cardiac output would increase to 10 L/min.
    D. Nothing; cardiac output is independent of heart rate.
    E. Cardiac output would triple.

1.64 Which ONE of the following statements is True regarding the term *blood pressure?*

    A. It is reported in cm H_2O unless otherwise specified.
    B. It represents the force exerted by the blood against any unit area of the vessel wall.
    C. It is constant throughout the cardiac cycle.
    D. It represents and can be used interchangeably with *flow.*
    E. It is the same as hydrostatic pressure.

1.65 The minimal pressure in the arterial system during a cardiac cycle is termed:

    A. Systolic pressure.
    B. Pulse pressure.
    C. Diastolic pressure.
    D. Mean pressure.
    E. Mean pulse pressure.

1.66 In measuring human blood pressure, the first sound was heard at 130 mmHg, the second at 105, the third at 100, and the last at 95. What is the estimated *mean* blood pressure?

    A. 118 mmHg.
    B. 115 mmHg.
    C. 122 mmHg.
    D. 107 mmHg.
    E. 104 mmHg.

1.67 Which ONE of the following is a correct statement describing transmission of the arterial pressure wave?

    A. It originates at the level of the arterioles.
    B. It slows with increasing age.
    C. It slows with increasing calcification of the vessels.
    D. It is caused in part by the inertia of blood in the aorta.

1.68 In laminar flow, the velocity of the blood is:

    A. Directly proportional to the cross-sectional area of the vessel.
    B. Lowest when kinetic energy is highest.
    C. Lowest at the center of the vessel.
    D. Zero at the vessel wall.
    E. Highest at the vessel wall.

1.69 The principal site of peripheral resistance in the vascular bed is determined to be in the arterioles because:

    A. The blood pressure does not change across these vessels.
    B. The blood flow is slowest in the arterioles.
    C. The pressure drop across these vessels is greatest.
    D. These vessels have thick muscular coats.
    E. The blood pressure is highest here.

1.70 As the arterial pressure wave moves toward the periphery, all of the following occur *except*:

    A. The pulse amplitude is increased by the presence of reflected waves.
    B. Speed of propagation diminishes.
    C. Pulsatile changes in arterioles and capillaries are "dampened" owing to vascular distensibility and resistance.
    D. Speed of propagation increases.

1.71 The incisura on the aortic pressure wave:

    A. Indicates closure of the AV valves.
    B. Occurs when the aortic valve opens.
    C. Is inscribed just after the aortic valve closes.
    D. Occurs during rapid ventricular filling.
    E. Result from aortic valve malfunction.

1.72 Starling's law of the heart can best be expressed by which one of the following?

    A. As heart rate increases, ventricular contractility also increases.
    B. Increasing the arterial pressure decreases the stroke volume.
    C. Within limits, an increase in venous return results in an increase in stroke volume.
    D. The product of heart rate and stroke volume equals the cardiac output.

1.73 Which ONE of the following best describes the role of the heart as a pump ?

    A. Regulating cardiac output.
    B. Forcing blood from the venous to the arterial circulation, restoring energy necessary for the blood flow.
    C. Suctioning blood from the venous circulation.
    D. Removing carbon dioxide from venous blood and supplying oxygen.

TWO

TECHNIQUE

2.0 Which ultrasound system control automatically calibrates for measurements?

    A. Overall gain.
    B. Reject.
    C. Near gain.
    D. Depth.

2.1 Increasing system gain can reduce technical artifacts.

    True or False

The purpose of the time-gain compensation (TGC) circuit is: (True or False)

    2.2 To suppress near-field echos.
    2.3 To enhance far-field echos.
    2.4 To selectively eliminate weak echos.
    2.5 To compensate for loss of ultrasound energy (attenuation) as the beam enters the body.

Which of the following are True/False regarding the side lobes seen in two-dimensional images?

> **2.6** They are generated from the edges of individual transducer elements.
> **2.7** They are a greater problem with mechanical systems.
> **2.8** They are a greater problem with phased-array systems.
> **2.9** They display fuzzy areas on the image.

In a parasternal long-axis transducer position, imaging is being done from the *wrong* intercostal space when: (True or False)

> **2.10** The interventricular septum and the anterior aortic root wall meet at a right angle.
> **2.11** The interventricular septum and the anterior aortic root wall are contiguous.
> **2.12** The interventricular septum and the anterior aortic root wall do not meet.
> **2.13** The interventricular septum and the posterior aortic root wall meet.

2.14 With which of the following conditions would a contrast agent *not* likely be used to enhance the echo diagnosis?

> A. Atrial septal defect.
> B. Idiopathic hypertrophic subaortic stenosis.
> C. Ventricular septal defect.
> D. Patent ductus arteriosus.

Left-to-right shunts are more difficult than right-to-left shunts to detect with peripheral-vein contrast injections because:

> **2.15** Contrast is totally filtered out at the pulmonary capillary level.
> **2.16** Negative contrast is not as easy to identify as positive contrast.
> **2.17** Microbubbles will not travel left to right because of pressure differences.
> **2.18** The microbubbles traveling from the right side into the left are rare and difficult to see.

2.19 In which condition could amyl nitrite be useful?

> A. Mitral stenosis.
> B. Atrial septal defect.
> C. Aortic stenosis.
> D. Idiopathic hypertrophic subaortic stenosis.

In the patient with hypertrophic obstructive cardiomyopathy (HOCM) with no systolic anterior motion (SAM) at rest, SAM may be demonstrated by the use of: (True or False)

2.20 The valsalva maneuver.
2.21 Amyl nitrite.
2.22 Inspiration.
2.23 Expiration.

When using a large sample volume in performing a Doppler examination, the operator: (True or False)

2.24 Lengthens the examination time.
2.25 Minimizes the chances of missing jets.
2.26 Increases the chances of erroneously detecting flow in adjacent chambers.
2.27 Reduces the sensitivity of the instrument.

2.28 The apical four-chamber view is frequently the first approach for a Doppler study because:

A. It is the easiest location from which to obtain image and Doppler information.
B. The transducer is closest to the valves in this position.
C. The Doppler beam is parallel to the flow through multiple valves.
D. More abnormalities can be identified from this location.

2.29 Parasternal long-axis views are good for Doppler applications because of the relationship of angle to flow.

True or False

THREE

EVALUATION OF THE MITRAL VALVE

3.0 Left atrial dilatation is associated with:

    A. Significant mitral regurgitation.
    B. Increased pulmonary pressures.
    C. Patent ductus arteriosus.
    D. All of the above.

3.1 The E–F slope of the mitral valve corresponds to which event in the cardiac cycle?

    A. The "conduit phase."
    B. Rapid diastolic filling.
    C. Early systole.
    D. Late systole.

The posterior leaflet of the mitral valve appears to have a smaller excursion than the anterior leaflet because: (True or False)

    3.2 It is intersected at an angle that does not show its full size.
    3.3 The leaflet never completely opens.
    3.4 Its excursion is smaller.
    3.5 The shape is different than that of the anterior leaflet.

Generally, the E–F slope of the mitral valve has been considered to provide a reliable assessment of: (True or False)

3.6 Left atrial enlargement.
3.7 Left atrial myxoma.
3.8 Mitral stenosis.
3.9 Left ventricular function.

An increase in the size of the A wave of the mitral valve suggests: (True or False)

3.10 Left ventricular enlargement.
3.11 Aortic insufficiency.
3.12 An increase in left ventricular end diastolic pressure.
3.13 Left ventricular hypokinesis.

3.14 Normal opening of the mitral valve is caused by the pressures being higher in the left ventricle than in the left atrium.

True or False

The mitral valve is composed of: (True or False)

3.15 Chordae tendineae.
3.16 Mitral annuli.
3.17 Fibrous bands.
3.18 Papillary muscles.

3.19 The M-mode criterion that defines mitral stenosis the *least* is:

A. Anterior movement of the posterior leaflet.
B. A reduced E–F slope.
C. An increased A–C interval.
D. A dense, thickened appearance of the valve.

3.20 The mitral two-dimensional echo view that best allows calculation of the mitral orifice is the:

    A. Parasternal long-axis view.
    B. Apical two-chamber view.
    C. Parasternal short-axis view.
    D. Subcostal four-chamber view.

Factors that influence the short-axis two-dimensional measurement of the mitral valve are: (True or False)

    3.21 The lateral resolution.
    3.22 Gain.
    3.23 Transducer frequency.
    3.24 The axial resolution.

The color-flow examination of the stenotic mitral valve would typically display: (True or False)

    3.25 A narrow jet.
    3.26 A central blue zone.
    3.27 A central red zone.
    3.28 Surrounding yellow and red hues.

3.29 The mitral two-dimensional echo view that is most used in continuous-wave Doppler imaging of mitral stenosis is the:

    A. Parasternal long-axis view.
    B. Apical four-chamber view.
    C. Parasternal short-axis view.
    D. Subcostal four-chamber view.

3.30 The criterion that is the most helpful in defining mitral stenosis is:

    A. Left ventricular enlargement.
    B. Left ventricular hypertrophy.
    C. Left atrial enlargement.
    D. Aortic root dilatation.

3.31 Following a mitral commissurotomy, the valve orifice can be accurately evaluated with the:

    A. M mode, by defining the leaflet separation.
    B. Two-dimensional echocardiography, by imaging the actual orifice.
    C. Doppler, by the velocity of the flow and Bernoulli's equation.
    D. Doppler, by estimating valve area using the pressure half-time formula.

3.32 Which of the following mitral conditions could cause mitral regurgitation?

    A. Mitral stenosis.
    B. Mitral prolapse.
    C. Mitral vegetation.
    D. All the above.

The aortic valve M-mode motion is often abnormal in patients with mitral regurgitation, demonstrating: (True or False)

    3.33 A flutter of the aortic leaflets in systole.
    3.34 Early systolic closure.
    3.35 Gradual closure during systole.
    3.36 All of the above.

The M-mode findings in mitral regurgitation are: (True or False)

    3.37 Left ventricular dilatation.
    3.38 Left atrial enlargement.
    3.39 Flutter of the interventricular septum.
    3.40 Flutter of the posterior aortic root.

3.41 Peak mitral regurgitant velocity tells the examiner:

    A. The severity of mitral regurgitation.
    B. Maximum instantaneous pressure difference between the left ventricle and left atrium.
    C. The cause of the mitral regurgitation.
    D. The direction of the regurgitant jet.

3.42 A two-dimensional echo criterion that can be very helpful in determining mitral regurgitation is:

    A. High-frequency oscillations of the mitral valve.
    B. Premature closure of the aortic valve.
    C. Left ventricular enlargement.
    D. Left ventricular hypertrophy.

3.43 The two-dimensional echo view best for Doppler analysis of mitral regurgitation is:

    A. The parasternal long-axis view.
    B. The parasternal short-axis view.
    C. The apical four-chamber view.
    D. None of the above.

3.44 Left atrial enlargement could be a criterion for determining mitral regurgitation.

    True or False

3.45 Mitral regurgitation is always associated with mitral valve prolapse.

    True or False

3.46 Which of the mitral conditions listed below could be associated with mitral regurgitation?

    A. Rupture of the chordae.
    B. Flail leaflet.
    C. Annular calcification.
    D. All of the above.
    E. None of the above.

The echo/Doppler findings in papillary muscle dysfunction are: (True or False)

    3.47 Left ventricular enlargement.
    3.48 Mitral regurgitation.
    3.49 Mitral annulus dilatation.
    3.50 Incomplete mitral valve closure.

3.51 The term *myxomatous degeneration* used to describe a mitral valve prolapse denotes:

    A. Thickening of the mitral valve leaflets.
    B. A myxoma in the vicinity of the mitral valve.
    C. Redundancy of the mitral valve leaflets.
    D. A vegetation on the mitral valve leaflets.

M-mode findings with a flail mitral valve are: (True or False)

    3.52 Fine systolic flutter of the mitral valve.
    3.53 Coarse, choatic diastolic flutter of the anterior or posterior mitral leaflet.
    3.54 Mitral leaflets noted in the left atrium during systole.
    3.55 Noncoaptation of the anterior and posterior mitral valve leaflets.

Doming of the anterior mitral leaflet is seen in: (True or False)

    3.56 Mitral stenosis.
    3.57 Redundant, floppy mitral valve.
    3.58 Flail mitral leaflet.
    3.59 Vegetation/mass involving free edge at the anterior leaflet.

3.60 Which set of echocardiographic features best predicts the presence of mitral stenosis in combined mitral stenosis and mitral insufficiency?

    A. Separation of the mital valve leaflets on the two-dimensional parasternal short-axis view.
    B. Doming on the two-dimensional parasternal long-axis view.
    C. Reduced E–F slope on the M mode.
    D. Thickened leaflets, seen on the apical four-chamber view.

Mitral annular calcification may obscure the: (True or False)

    3.61 Anterior mitral valve leaflet.
    3.62 Posterior mitral valve leaflet.
    3.63 Endocardial echoes.
    3.64 Epicardial echoes.

Mitral and tricuspid regurgitation are easily differentiated by Doppler because of: (True or False)

    3.65 Differences in timing of valve opening and closing.

    3.66 Different locations of the jets.

    3.67 Different directions of the jets.

    3.68 Differences in forward flow velocity curves.

3.69 The normal brief posterior displacement of the interventricular septum with the onset of diastole (diastolic dip) may be exaggerated in:

    A. Mitral insufficiency.

    B. Mitral stenosis.

    C. Aortic insufficiency.

    D. Aortic stenosis.

Common echo-Doppler findings in patients with Marfan's syndrome are: (True or False)

    3.70 Aortic root dilatation.

    3.71 Mitral valve prolapse.

    3.72 Pulmonary insufficiency.

    3.73 Aortic regurgitation.

Mitral leaflet motion is influenced by: (True or False)

    3.74 The relative pressures in the left atrium and left ventricle.

    3.75 The velocity and volume of blood flow through the mitral orifice.

    3.76 Left ventricular diastolic compliance.

    3.77 Systolic performance of the left ventricle.

3.78 In the M-mode recording of mitral stenosis, the posterior leaflet of the mitral valve moves anteriorly with the anterior leaflet:

    A. Always.

    B. In 80 to 90% of cases.

    C. In 30 to 40% of cases.

    D. Never.

A reduced E–F slope of the mitral valve on M mode is seen with: (True or False)

> **3.79** Aortic valve disease.
> **3.80** Reduced left ventricular compliance.
> **3.81** Mitral stenosis.
> **3.82** Dilated cardiomyopathy.

Two-dimensional determination of the size of a stenotic mitral orifice is optimal only if: (True or False)

> **3.83** Viewed in the parasternal short axis.
> **3.84** Gain settings are carefully set.
> **3.85** Doming of the anterior mitral leaflet is observed.
> **3.86** The scan plane is parallel to and passes directly through the valve orifice.

FOUR

EVALUATION OF THE AORTIC VALVE

4.0 Aortic valve closure is related to an increased pressure in the aorta relative to the left ventricle.

True or False

4.1 The amplitude of aortic root motion has been used to assess:

A. The vigor of left ventricular contraction.
B. The degree of aortic stenosis.
C. The degree of aortic insufficiency.
D. The size of the left atrium.

4.2 Findings consistent with aortic stenosis seen on the M-mode echocardiogram include:

A. Normal thickness of the left ventricular wall.
B. Thickened aortic leaflets.
C. A dilated left atrium.
D. Hyperdynamic left ventricular contractility.

4.3 The M-mode findings of a young patient with congenital aortic stenosis frequently demonstrate:

    A. Systolic doming of the cusps.
    B. Normal leaflet separation.
    C. Thickened, restricted cusps.
    D. Diastolic separation of the cusps.

Aortic insufficiency can alter the motion or appearance of the mitral valve by: (True or False)

    4.4 Fluttering the leaflets in diastole.
    4.5 Reducing the closing velocity of the mitral leaflets.
    4.6 Producing shaggy echoes around the mitral valve.
    4.7 Decreasing cusp separation.

Similar spectral patterns can be seen with aortic insufficiency and mitral stenosis. The best way(s) to differentiate the two when both are present is/are to: (True or False)

    4.8 Be aware that aortic insufficiency will have a less intense signal than mitral stenosis.
    4.9 Rotate the patient more laterally.
    4.10 Use the smallest feasible sample volume and carefully evaluate the area.
    4.11 Use continuous-wave Doppler from the suprasternal notch.

4.12 The M-mode criterion that is *not* useful for defining aortic stenosis is:

    A. Dense, thick aortic valve echoes.
    B. A reduced "box" opening.
    C. Diastolic aortic valve oscillation.
    D. Left ventricular hypertrophy.

4.13 The best two-dimensional view used for imaging and calculating the aortic valve orifice is the:

    A. Parasternal long-axis view.
    B. Parasternal short-axis view.
    C. Apical four-chamber view.
    D. Apical two-chamber view.

4.14 The best approach for continuous-wave Doppler analysis of aortic stenosis is the:

    A. Parasternal.
    B. Apical.
    C. Suprasternal.
    D. Subcostal.

4.15 Overestimation of Doppler peak gradients in aortic stenosis occur with coexistent:

    A. Aortic insufficiency.
    B. Mitral stenosis.
    C. Mitral regurgitation.
    D. Tricuspid regurgitation.

The Doppler formula $4 \times (V_2{}^2 - V_1{}^2)$ is important in: (True or False)

    4.16 Aortic stenosis.
    4.17 Mitral regurgitation.
    4.18 Left ventricular outflow tract obstruction.
    4.19 Mitral stenosis.

In patients with aortic stenosis and low peak velocity due to poor left ventricular function (low flow state), the continuous-wave Doppler waveform should be analyzed for: (True or False)

    4.20 Time to peak velocity.
    4.21 Shape of the spectral waveform.
    4.22 Mean velocity.
    4.23 Intensity of signal.

High velocity recorded below the baseline on the Doppler spectrum when imaging from the apex by continuous-wave Doppler could be related to: (True or False)

    4.24 Aortic stenosis.
    4.25 Aortic regurgitation.
    4.26 Mitral regurgitation.
    4.27 Left ventricular outflow tract obstruction.

4.28 The criterion that is *not* helpful for defining aortic stenosis is:

    A. Left ventricular hypertrophy.
    B. Aortic postvalvular dilatation.
    C. Left ventricular enlargement.
    D. Diastolic oscillations of the aortic cusps.

4.29 Bicuspid aortic stenosis is a congenital abnormality.

    True or False

4.30 Valve mobility may be the most helpful factor in defining the difference between aortic stenosis and sclerosis.

    True or False

4.31 Aortic regurgitation can best be defined by the M-mode criterion of:

    A. High-frequency oscillations of the aortic valve.
    B. Left ventricular hypertrophy.
    C. Aortic root dilatation.
    D. High-frequency oscillations of the mitral valve.

4.32 One of the first indications of aortic regurgitation noted by two-dimensional echo is:

    A. Left atrial enlargement.
    B. Thickened aortic valve.
    C. Left ventricular hypertrophy.
    D. Left ventricular enlargement.

4.33 Aortic regurgitation is best evaluated by Doppler in the:

    A. Parasternal long-axis view.
    B. Parasternal short-axis view.
    C. Apical four-chamber view.
    D. Subcostal four-chamber view.

4.34 Paradoxical septal motion is most commonly associated with aortic regurgitation.

True or False

4.35 Aortic regurgitation may be associated with bacterial endocarditis of the aortic valve.

True or False

Color flow examinations of the aortic valve flow in patients with aortic stenosis should be performed from which view: (True or False)

4.36 High right parasternal.
4.37 High left parasternal.
4.38 Apical.
4.39 Suprasternal notch.

The Doppler recording can underestimate aortic stenosis peak velocity if: (True or False)

4.40 There is reduced cardiac output.
4.41 There is associated aortic regurgitation.
4.42 The maximum jet is not recorded.
4.43 The angle of incidence is greater than 20°.

4.44 Early closure of the mitral valve in patients with acute aortic insufficiency is due to:

A. Reduced cardiac output.
B. The regurgitant jet restricting mitral valve motion.
C. Elevated left ventricular diastolic pressure.
D. Reduced left ventricular compliance.

The effect of aortic regurgitation on the left ventricle is: (True or False)

4.45 Concentric left ventricular hypertrophy.
4.46 Increased septal motion.
4.47 Left ventricular dilatation.
4.48 Septal flutter.

The M-mode findings in patients with aortic regurgitation may include: (True or False)

      4.49 Fine systolic flutter of the aortic cusps.
      4.50 Fine diastolic flutter of the aortic cusps.
      4.51 Diastolic echoes in the left ventricular outflow tract.
      4.52 Systolic flutter of the interventricular septum.

4.53 Reverse doming of the anterior mitral valve leaflet can be observed in:

      A. Idiopathic hypertrophic subaortic stenosis.
      B. Aortic stenosis.
      C. Aortic regurgitation.
      D. Mitral regurgitation.

Methods used in quantitating the severity of aortic insufficiency are: (True or False)

      4.54 Mapping the flow disturbance with a pulsed-wave system.
      4.55 Taking the peak velocity of regurgitation, using a continuous-wave Doppler system, and putting it into the modified Bernoulli equation $(4V^2)$.
      4.56 Calculating the pressure half-time from the continuous-wave Doppler waveform.
      4.57 Using color-flow imaging to evaluate thickness of the regurgitant stream at its origin.

In combined aortic stenosis and aortic insufficiency, the continuous-wave aortic waveform must be carefully analyzed so that the severity of the aortic stenosis will be correctly assessed. A mild gradient may be expected if: (True or False)

      4.58 A high peak velocity is recorded with an early-peaking, asymmetrical, rapidly descending spectrum.
      4.59 A high peak velocity is recorded with a later-peaking, symmetrical spectrum.
      4.60 A low peak velocity is recorded with a late-peaking, symmetrical waveform.
      4.61 A low peak velocity is recorded with early-peaking, asymmetrical waveform.

FIVE

EVALUATION OF THE TRICUSPID VALVE

5.0 Tricuspid valve hemodynamics occur approximately 50 milliseconds prior to mitral valve hemodynamics.

True or False

The M-mode criteria for tricuspid stenosis includes the following: (True or False)

5.1 Dense, thick leaflets.
5.2 A reduced E–F slope.
5.3 A reduced A wave.
5.4 An increased A wave.

The two-dimensional echo views that allow visualization of at least two tricuspid leaflets include: (True or False)

5.5 Parasternal long-axis (right heart).
5.6 Parasternal short-axis.
5.7 Apical four-chamber.
5.8 Apical.

5.9 The best two-dimensional echo view for Doppler analysis of the tricuspid valve is the:

    A. Parasternal long-axis view.
    B. Parasternal short-axis view.
    C. Apical four-chamber view.
    D. Suprasternal long-axis view.

5.10 Which condition is most indicative of tricuspid stenosis?

    A. Right ventricular enlargement.
    B. Right ventricular hypertrophy.
    C. Right atrial enlargement.
    D. Pulmonary insufficiency.

5.11 Which tricuspid M-mode criterion clearly indicates tricuspid regurgitation?

    A. Reduced E–F slope.
    B. Mid to late prolapse.
    C. Notching.
    D. None of the above.

5.12 Which of the following two-dimensional echo criteria may be most useful in defining tricuspid regurgitation?

    A. Reduced tricuspid E–F slope.
    B. Right ventricular enlargement.
    C. Right ventricular hypertrophy.
    D. Right atrial enlargement.

5.13 The two-dimensional echo view that is best for Doppler analysis of tricuspid regurgitation is the:

    A. Parasternal long-axis view.
    B. Parasternal short-axis view.
    C. Apical four-chamber view.
    D. Suprasternal long-axis view.

5.14 Bacterial endocarditis most commonly occurs on the:

    A. Mitral valve.
    B. Tricuspid valve.
    C. Aortic valve.
    D. Pulmonic valve.

Echocardiographic features of carcinoid heart disease involving the tricuspid valve are: (True or False)

    5.15 Tricuspid regurgitation.
    5.16 Tricuspid prolapse.
    5.17 Thickened, immobile leaflets.
    5.18 Increased pressure half-time.

When performing a Doppler examination of the inferior vena cava and/or hepatic veins for evidence of tricuspid regurgitation, one would expect to find: (True or False)

    5.19 Flow toward the transducer in systole.
    5.20 Flow away from the transducer in systole.
    5.21 Flow toward the transducer in diastole.
    5.22 Flow away from the transducer in diastole.

5.23 Tricuspid regurgitation can be recognized on an M-mode study of the inferior vena cava in which contrast medium is injected into an arm vein by the appearance of contrast medium:

    A. Following atrial systole.
    B. During ventricular systole.
    C. Following atrial diastole.
    D. During ventricular diastole.

Tricuspid inflow velocity normally resembles mitral inflow except: (True or False)

    5.24 Tricuspid valve inflow is at a higher velocity.
    5.25 Tricuspid valve inflow is at a lower velocity.
    5.26 Tricuspid valve inflow increases with inspiration.
    5.27 Tricuspid valve inflow decreases with inspiration.

Significant tricuspid regurgitation is present on the Doppler two-dimensional examination when: (True or False)

    5.28 Localized tricuspid regurgitation signals are noted.
    5.29 Right atrial dimension is increased.
    5.30 Systolic flow into the hepatic veins is observed in the subcostal approach.
    5.31 The tricuspid regurgitation jet hugs the interatrial septum.

Doppler features of tricuspid stenosis include: (True or False)

    5.32 An increase in peak velocity.
    5.33 A slow rate of descent of the velocity curve following peak velocity.
    5.34 A decrease in velocity with inspiration.
    5.35 Diastolic dispersion.

5.36 Tricuspid regurgitation peak velocity is proportional to the:

    A. Diastolic pressure gradient between the right ventricle and right atrium.
    B. Systolic pressure gradient between the right ventricle and right atrium.
    C. Diastolic pressure gradient between the right ventricle and the pulmonary artery.
    D. Systolic pressure gradient between the right ventricle and the pulmonary artery.

5.37 During a contrast study, contrast appearing in the inferior vena cava and hepatic veins during right ventricular systole indicates:

    A. Tricuspid stenosis.
    B. Tricuspid insufficiency.
    C. Pulmonary hypertension.
    D. Pulmonary insufficiency.

The differences in timing of the opening and closing of the mitral valve and tricuspid valves are: (True or False)

    5.38. Tricuspid valve closure occurs prior to mitral valve closure.
    5.39. Tricuspid valve closure occurs after mitral valve closure.
    5.40. Tricuspid valve opening occurs prior to mitral valve opening.
    5.41. Tricuspid valve opening occurs after mitral valve opening.

5.42 The parasternal long-axis right ventricular inflow view demonstrates which tricuspid valve leaflets?

    A. Anterior and septal.
    B. Anterior and posterior.
    C. Septal and posterior.
    D. Inferior and posterior.

To distinguish the tricuspid valve from the mitral valve when attempting to identify the morphology of the right ventricle, one looks for: (True or False)

    5.43 More apical insertion of the septal leaflet of the tricuspid valve (in relation to the anterior mitral leaflet).
    5.44 More basal insertion of the septal leaflet of the tricuspid valve (in relation to the anterior mitral leaflet).
    5.45 The trileaflet configuration of the tricuspid valve.
    5.46 The presence of four distinct papillary muscles.

Tricuspid valve echo findings in patients with such acquired diseases as endomyocardial fibrosis, endocardial fibroelastosis, and malignant carcinoid include: (True or False)

    5.47 Increased E to A ratio.
    5.48 Thickened leaflets and chordae.
    5.49 Diastolic leaflet doming.
    5.50 Restriction of leaflet motion.

The most reliable views for demonstrating doming of the stenotic tricuspid valve are: (True or False)

    5.51 Parasternal long-axis, right ventricular inflow.
    5.52 Parasternal short-axis.
    5.53 Apical four-chamber.
    5.54 All of the above.

Signs of right ventricular volume overload in tricuspid regurgitation include: (True or False)

5.55 Dilatation of the right ventricle.

5.56 Dilatation of the right atrium.

5.57 Flattening of the septum during diastole.

5.58 Anterior motion of the interventricular septum during isovolumetric contraction.

SIX

EVALUATION OF THE PULMONIC VALVE

6.0 The most superior and lateral cardiac valve is the:

    A. Mitral valve.
    B. Tricuspid valve.
    C. Aortic valve.
    D. Pulmonic valve.

6.1 M-mode recordings of the pulmonic valve normally show which of the pulmonary leaflets?

    A. Right.
    B. Left.
    C. Posterior.

6.2 The pulmonic valve may not be visualized in which two-dimensional echo view?

    A. Parasternal short-axis.
    B. Subcostal short-axis.
    C. Apical four-chamber.

6.3 Pulsed Doppler recordings of pulmonary insufficiency are normally recorded in the:

    A. Parasternal long-axis view.
    B. Parasternal short-axis view.
    C. Suprasternal long-axis view.
    D. Apical two-chamber view.

6.4 Pulmonic regurgitation may occur in:

    A. In bacterial endocarditis.
    B. In pulmonary hypertension.
    C. After a pulmonary valvotomy.
    D. All of the above.

Characteristic findings on the two-dimensional echo of the pulmonic valve in pulmonary stenosis include: (True or False)

    6.5 Leaflet tips that remain centrally located in systole.
    6.6 Doming of the leaflets in systole.
    6.7 Eversion of the leaflets in diastole.
    6.8 Thickening of the leaflets.

The right ventricular outflow tract can be divided into the: (True or False)

    6.9   Midvalvular level.
    6.10 Infundibular level.
    6.11 Valvular level.
    6.12 Supravalvular level.

To differentiate significant pulmonary insufficiency from "normal" pulmonary insufficiency, one should look for: (True or False)

    6.13 Disturbed flow distal to the valve.
    6.14 Associated signs of pulmonary hypertension.
    6.15 Diffuse distribution of regurgitation.
    6.16 Increased intensity of the continuous-wave Doppler waveform.

Acquired pulmonary regurgitation may be secondary to: (True or False)

    6.17 Pulmonary hypertension.
    6.18 Pacemaker wire.
    6.19 Bacterial endocarditis.
    6.20 Pulmonary valulotomy.

The pulmonic Doppler-flow pattern in pulmonary insufficiency secondary to pulmonary hypertension shows: (True or False)

    6.21 High-velocity disturbed flow throughout diastole.
    6.22 Short acceleration time.
    6.23 High-velocity disturbed flow throughout systole.
    6.24 A decrease in flow in midsystole.

6.25 Characteristic findings on the M-mode examination of the pulmonic valve in patients with pulmonary stenosis include:

    A. An exaggerated A wave.
    B. Doming.
    C. Absent A wave.
    D. Notching (early closure).

6.26 In comparison with normal flow-velocity acceleration time in the aortic valve, acceleration in the pulmonic valve is normally:

    A. Faster.
    B. The same.
    C. Not consistent.
    D. Slower.

Pulmonary regurgitation, which can cause right ventricular volume overload, may be manifested by: (True or False)

    6.27 Dilatation of the right ventricle.
    6.28 Abnormal septal motion.
    6.29 Flutter of the tricuspid valve leaflets.
    6.30 Dilatation of the right atrium.

The following are seen with pulmonary hypertension: (True or False)

6.31 Midsystolic notching of the A wave.
6.32 Nonvariation in A-wave amplitude.
6.33 Absence of the A wave.
6.34 Absence of the P wave.

SEVEN

EVALUATION
FOR
ENDOCARDITIS

7.0 The ability of M mode and two-dimensional echo to visualize vegetations is a useful and significant application of echocardiography.

True or False

Vegetations have been seen echocardiographically at sites other than on the valves. These sites include: (True or False)

7.1 Aneurysm of the sinus of Valsalva.
7.2 Calcified mitral annulus.
7.3 Infected ventricular septal defect.
7.4 Left atrial appendage.

7.5 Valve motion in endocarditis is:

A. Eccentric.
B. Exaggerated.
C. Reduced.
D. Normal.

Two-dimensional echo assists in evaluating the mitral valve in endocarditis by detecting associated: (True or False)

7.6 Flail mitral valve leaflets.
7.7 Left atrial thrombosis.
7.8 Ruptured chordae tendineae.
7.9 Mitral valve prolapse.

Predisposing factors for endocarditis of the aortic valve include: (True or False)

7.10 Intravenous drug abuse.
7.11 Rheumatic deformity of the valve.
7.12 Bicuspid aortic valve.
7.13 Calcification of aortic cusps in the elderly.

Imaging of vegetations is best attempted using the two-dimensional echo method because it defines: (True or False)

7.14 The type of infection.
7.15 The size of the vegetation.
7.16 The pattern of motion.
7.17 Location relative to other cardiac structures.

Mitral valve M-mode findings in endocarditis include: (True or False)

7.18 Leaflet separation in systole.
7.19 An abnormal mass of echoes on the valve leaflet.
7.20 Unobstructed motion of the valve leaflets.
7.21 Eccentric motion from beat to beat.

Vegetations from endocarditis may: (True or False)

7.22 Erode and disrupt the valve leaflets and adjacent structures.
7.23 Obstruct flow through the valve.
7.24 Dislodge, causing peripheral embolization.
7.25 Disappear with no adverse effect.

Complications secondary to endocarditis noted echocardiographically include: (True or False)

7.26 Fistula.
7.27 Myxoma.
7.28 Aneurysm.
7.29 Abscess.

Echocardiography is *not* the procedure of choice to diagnose endocarditis because: (True or False)

7.30 Not enough research has been performed to substantiate use of the technique.
7.31 It cannot differentiate new from old vegetations.
7.32 It cannot identify vegetations smaller than 2 mm.
7.33 The results are rarely definitive.

EIGHT

EVALUATION OF PROSTHETIC VALVES

8.0 The most common problem associated with prosthetic valves is:

    A. Strut fracture.
    B. Improper seating.
    C. Clotting problems.
    D. Disk fracture.

8.1 Quantitation of prosthetic-valve motion is best accomplished by:

    A. M-mode scanning.
    B. Two-dimensional scanning.
    C. Doppler ultrasound.
    D. Magnetic resonance imaging (MRI).

8.2 The Starr-Edwards ball prosthesis has the following number of orifices:

    A. One.
    B. Two.
    C. Three.
    D. Four.
    E. Five.

All prosthetic valves are inherently restrictive. Therefore, when evaluating a prosthetic valve for stenosis, one must take into account not only the velocity of blood flow but also: (True or False)

> 8.3 Valve size.
> 8.4 Patient size.
> 8.5 The age of the valve.
> 8.6 Cardiac output.

A mechanical prosthesis that reveals incomplete or delayed opening on the M-mode echo suggests: (True or False)

> 8.7   Deterioration of the valve.
> 8.8   Swelling of the valve.
> 8.9   Thrombus on the valve.
> 8.10 Dehiscence of the valve.

A Doppler recording from a stenotic mitral bioprosthesis might include: (True or False)

> 8.11 A rapid diminution in diastolic velocity.
> 8.12 High peak velocity.
> 8.13 Slow diminution in diastolic velocity.
> 8.14 Turbulent flow.

Higher than normal maximum velocities recorded in a prosthetic valve may be seen with associated: (True or False)

> 8.15 Increased left ventricular end-diastolic pressure.
> 8.16 Transprosthetic or paraprosthetic regurgitation.
> 8.17 Congestive heart failure.
> 8.18 Increased cardiac output.

The best approach(es) for obtaining the highest velocity in an aortic prosthesis is/are from the: (True or False)

> 8.19 Left parasternal view.
> 8.20 Apex.
> 8.21 Suprasternal notch.
> 8.22 Right sternal border.

Continuous-wave Doppler is the Doppler technique of choice in measuring transprosthetic blood flow velocities because: (True or False)

8.23 It enables the operator to localize the peak velocity.
8.24 It ensures registration of the peak velocity.
8.25 Prosthetic valves are often stenotic and produce increased velocities.
8.26 It is easier to record the flow velocities with continuous-wave Doppler.

Abnormalities of the bioprosthetic valve seen on echocardiography include: (True or False)

8.27 Excessive rocking motion of the valve apparatus.
8.28 Increased leaflet thickness.
8.29 A focal mass of echoes attached to the valve leaflets.
8.30 Shadowing of the struts and sewing rings.

Mechanical prosthetic valves include: (True or False)

8.31 Ball in cage.
8.32 Disk in cage.
8.33 Tilting disk.
8.34 Double tilting disk.

Bioprosthetic leaflet thickening observed on the echo can be associated with: (True or False)

8.35 Valvular stenosis.
8.36 Infectious endocarditis.
8.37 Normal prosthesis function.
8.38 Peripheral embolization.

8.39 All three struts of the aortic or mitral bioprosthesis can be seen when imaged from the:

A. Parasternal long-axis view.
B. Parasternal short-axis view.
C. Apical four-chamber view.
D. Subcostal four-chamber view.

8.40 Mitral prosthetic valvular dehiscence is demonstrated on echocardiography by:

    A. Valve leaflet echoes appearing in the left atrium in systole.
    B. Rocking, erratic motion of the valve apparatus.
    C. Thickened appearance of the valve apparatus.
    D. A bright, focal mass on one valve leaflet.

8.41 Rounding of the E point detected by M mode in a Bjork-Shiley mechanical prosthesis in the mitral or tricuspid position indicates:

    A. Normal function of the valve.
    B. Regurgitation of the valve.
    C. Obstruction of the valve.
    D. A flail leaflet.

NINE

EVALUATION FOR PERICARDITIS

9.0 With M mode, constrictive pericarditis is best identified by a:

    A. Rapid early mitral E–F slope.
    B. Reduced left ventricular posterior wall amplitude.
    C. Flattening of mid to late left ventricular posterior wall motion.
    D. Reduced interventricular septal amplitude.

9.1 Echocardiography free spaces noted anteriorly but not posteriorly should always be considered pericardial effusions.

    True or False

Of the following, which is/are echo criteria for cardiac tamponade? (True or False)

    9.2 An increase in right ventricular size with inspiration.
    9.3 Posterior motion of the anterior right ventricular wall in diastole.
    9.4 Early diastolic indention of the right ventricle.
    9.5 Flattening of the mitral E–F slope.

9.6 The differentiation between pleural effusion and pericardial effusion *cannot* be assisted by:

    A. A double echo-free space posterior to the left ventricle.
    B. An anterior echo-free space.
    C. A paradoxical septal motion.
    D. A scan from apex to base.

Pitfalls to be avoided when looking for pericardial effusions with M mode include: (True or False)

    9.7 Setting gain too high.
    9.8 Mistaking the descending aorta.
    9.9 Directing the beam too lateral and picking up reverberations.
    9.10 Noting anterior echo-free space only.

The characteristics used to distinguish between pericardial fat and pericardial effusion are: (True or False)

    9.11 The density of echoes.
    9.12 Consistent distance between the pericardium and epicardium throughout the cardiac cycle.
    9.13 A distance greater than 2 mm between the pericardium and the epicardium.
    9.14 Anterior motion of the left ventricular pulmonary wedge pericardium during systole.

TEN

EVALUATION FOR CARDIOMYOPATHY

10.0 The appearance of left atrial myxoma on M mode mimics what other condition commonly seen with M mode?

    A. Ruptured sinus of Valsalva.
    B. Cor triatriatum.
    C. Mitral stenosis.
    D. Flail leaflet.

10.1 Of the following, which is *not* a criterion for idiopathic hypertrophic subaortic stenosis (IHSS)?

    A. Asymmetric septal hypertrophy.
    B. Midsystolic A-V notching.
    C. Systolic anterior motion of the mitral valve.
    D. High-frequency oscillations of the mitral valve.

10.2 Symmetrical hypokinesis is a differentiating echo feature for:

    A. Ischemic heart disease.
    B. Hypertrophic cardiomyopathy.
    C. Dilated cardiomyopathy.
    D. Congenital aortic stenosis.

10.3 Systolic anterior motion (SAM) is most commonly associated with which of these conditions?

    A. Left ventricular aneurysm.
    B. Left atrial myxoma.
    C. Idiopathic hypertrophic subaortic stenosis (IHSS).
    D. Aortic insufficiency.

10.4 Right ventricular volume overload (RVVO) is associated with the septal motions of:

    A. Diastolic "double dip."
    B. Anterior motion in early systole.
    C. Anterior motion in late systole.
    D. Akinesis.

10.5 The motion of the interventricular septum typically noted in left bundle branch block (LBBB) is:

    A. "Beaking."
    B. Paradoxical.
    C. Flat.
    D. Hyperkinetic.

An increase in E-point septal separation is used to evaluate: (True or False)

    10.6 Left ventricular function.
    10.7 Aneurysms.
    10.8 Left ventricular dilatation.
    10.9 Right ventricular infarction.

ELEVEN

ISCHEMIC HEART DISEASE AND MISCELLANEOUS DISORDERS

11.0 Echocardiography is not useful for the detection of coronary artery disease.

True or False

11.1 The electrical aberration that would produce a sawtooth pattern in an M-mode scan of a mitral valve is:

    A. A left bundle branch block (LBBB).
    B. A right bundle branch block (RBBB).
    C. The Wolff-Parkinson-White (WPW) syndrome.
    D. Atrial fibrillation.

Early systolic "beaking" of the interventricular septum is noted on M mode with: (True or False)

    11.2 Right bundle branch block.
    11.3 Left bundle branch block.
    11.4 Electrical pacing.
    11.5 Type B Wolff-Parkinson-White syndrome.

11.6 Atherosclerosis is a disease that begins in the:

    A. Adventitia.
    B. Intima.
    C. Transverse fibers.
    D. Inner media.
    E. Outer media.

Which of the following is/are true regarding atherosclerosis? (True or False)

    11.7 Atherosclerosis is a specific disease.
    11.8 Atherosclerosis usually develops at bifurcations.
    11.9 Atherosclerosis is a segmental disease.
    11.10 Atherosclerosis is a generalized disease.
    11.11 Intimal damage/repair may begin in adolescence.

11.12 In pathogenesis of thromboembolism, which of the following is likely to occur first?

    A. A loss of intimal continuity.
    B. Aggregation of platelets and fibrin.
    C. Fibrinoplatelet embolic shower.
    D. Development of fibrosis.
    E. Plaque hemorrhage.

11.13 Which of the following is *not* considered a risk factor for atherosclerosis?

    A. Hypertension.
    B. Being female.
    C. Diabetes mellitus.
    D. Lipoprotein abnormalities.
    E. Tobacco use.

TWELVE

CONGENITAL DISORDERS OF THE HEART

12.0 The interatrial septum is a thin, muscular membrane that separates the right and left atrial chambers. Echocardiographically it is best visualized in the following planes:

A. Apical four-chamber, subcostal long-axis, high right parasternal long-axis.
B. Apical four-chamber view, parasternal long- and short-axis view.
C. Subcostal long-axis and high parasternal short-axis views at the aortic level.
D. Apical four-chamber view, subcostal long-axis view, and parasternal short-axis view, at the aortic level.

12.1 The depression on the interatrial septum, termed the fossa ovalis, may be mistaken for an atrial septal defect if the correct window is not used; therefore the fossa ovalis area should be examined from the:

A. Apical window.
B. Subcostal window.
C. Parasternal short-axis window.
D. Subcostal short-axis window.

Changes in the orientation and shape of the interatrial septum are seen as the volume and pressure change within the atria.

12.2 With normal atrial pressures, the interatrial septum bows toward the right atrium.

True or False

12.3 As the left atrial volume increases, the interatrial septum bows more prominently toward the left atrium.

True or False

12.4 In chronic left atrial dilatation, the interatrial septum bows toward the left atrium during diastole and systole.

True or False

12.5 Right atrial volume overload causes the interatrial septum to bow toward the left atrium.

True or False

12.6 Excluding a bicuspid aortic valve, the most common congenital cardiac lesion that can be documented by echo in early adulthood is:

    A. Ventricular septal defect.
    B. Atrial septal defect.
    C. Mitral valve prolapse.
    D. Endocardial cushion defect.

12.7 Atrial septal defects are classified on the basis of their position in the septum and their embryologic origin. The most common is the:

    A. Ostium primum defect, located in the region of the fossa ovalis.
    B. Ostium primum defect, located near the base of the heart at the junction of the superior vena cava.
    C. Ostium secundum defect, located in the region of the fossa ovalis.
    D. Sinus venosus defect, located in the lower portion of the septum in continuity with the atrioventricular valves.

12.8 The most common echocardiographic features of an atrial septal defect are:

    A. Right ventricular volume overload, paradoxical septal motion, right-to-left shunting, septal brightness, and broadening at the edges of the defect.

    B. Increased right ventricular pressure overload, paradoxical septal motion, right-to-left shunting, mitral valve prolapse.

    C. Right ventricular volume overload, paradoxical septal motion, left-to-right shunting, broadening at the edges of the septum near an imaged defect.

    D. Decreased right ventricular pressure, right ventricular volume overload, normal septal motion, noncompliant left ventricle.

The interventricular septum is a thick, triangular muscular wall that separates the right and left ventricles. It may be visualized in several planes. The following planes are best suited for particular cardiac lesions:

12.9 The parasternal short-axis view is useful for recording defects in the region of the atrioventricular canal.

    True or False

12.10 The subcostal long-axis view is useful for visualizing defects in the muscular portion of the septum.

    True or False

12.11 The thickness of the septum as compared with the posterior heart wall is best visualized and measured in the apical four-chamber view.

    True or False

12.12 The parasternal short-axis view is most useful for visualizing membranous interventricular septal aneurysms.

    True or False

12.13 The most common congenital malformation of the heart is:

    A. Atrial septal defect.
    B. Tetralogy of Fallot.
    C. Ventricular septal defect.
    D. Transposition of the great arteries.

12.14 Ventricular septal defects are conventionally divided at the level of the crista supraventricularis into supracristal and infracristal.

True or False

12.15 The supracristal defects lie immediately below the aortic valve, with the valve forming the superior margin of the defect.

True or False

12.16 The most common ventricular septal defect is the muscular type.

True or False

12.17 Membranous defects may arise anywhere in the septum and may be small, large, or multiple.

True or False

12.18 Clinically, a large septal defect is more significant than multiple small defects.

True or False

12.19 Aortic valve overriding of the septum always occurs in the presence of a membranous ventricular septal defect.

True or False

12.20 The structure that plays a significant embryologic role in the development of the septum primum, atrioventricular valves, and membranous septum is the:

    A. Endocardial cushions.
    B. Ventral septal endocardium.
    C. Atrial septal endocardium.
    D. Endocardial fibroelastocushion.

12.21 Aortic valve prolapse is more likely to be visualized echocardiographically in the presence of:

    A. An aneurysm of the sinus of Valsalva.
    B. Rheumatic heart disease.
    C. A high perimembranous ventricular septal defect.
    D. A supracristal ventricular septal defect.
    E. A, C, and D.

12.22 In supravalvular aortic stenosis, localized or diffuse narrowing of the vessel is seen distal to the coronary arteries. This is most likely caused by:

    A. Hypoplasia of the ascending aorta.
    B. Bicuspid aortic valve.
    C. Marfan's syndrome.
    D. Fibrous membranous diaphragm above the aortic valve.
    E. A and D.

12.23 A high-pitched positive Doppler flow in diastole with the sample volume placed in the main pulmonary artery near the left-sided bifurcation most likely represents:

    A. A ventricular septal defect.
    B. Pulmonary insufficiency.
    C. Patent ductus arteriosus.
    D. Pulmonary stenosis.

12.24 Echographically the most common findings in a patient with tetralogy of Fallot are:

    A. Bicuspid aortic valve, hypoplasia of the aorta, ventricular septal defect, left ventricular hypertrophy.

    B. Subaortic ventricular septal defect, aortic overriding, right ventricular pressure overload, pulmonary stenosis.

    C. Muscular septal defect, aortic stenosis, left ventricular hypertrophy, right ventricular hypertrophy.

    D. Muscular ventricular septal defect, pulmonary stenosis, right ventricular volume overload, atrial septal defect.

12.25 Discrete subaortic stenosis is one form of left ventricular outflow tract obstruction. Echographically one would see:

    A. Discrete subaortic membrane, bicuspid aortic valve, left ventricular hypertrophy.

    B. Discrete subaortic membrane, poststenotic dilatation, left ventricular hypertrophy.

    C. Discrete subaortic membrane, left ventricular hypertrophy, thickened aortic valve with fluttering.

    D. Fibrous supraortic membrane, left ventricular hypertrophy, aortic stenosis.

12.26 Which of the following statements is *false* regarding coarctation of the aorta?

    A. The aortic constriction is due to a shelf of tissue arising from the posterolateral aspect of the aorta and projecting into the aortic lumen toward the ductal attachment.

    B. Frequently some degree of tubular hypoplasia of the aortic isthmus is present.

    C. Associated anomalies include patent ductus arteriosus, aortic stenosis, ventricular septal defect, and mitral valve abnormalities.

    D. Most aortic coarctations are at or below the diaphragm.

12.27 Transposition refers to a cardiac condition with the following problems:

A. Ventricular septal defect, patent ductus arteriosus, right-sided aortic arch, dextrocardia.
B. Pulmonary artery located posterior and to the left as it arises from the left ventricle; aortic valve anterior and to the right as it arises from the right ventricle.
C. Pulmonary artery arises from the infundibular portion of the right ventricular; aorta arises from the outlet portion of the right ventricle.
D. Atria are located on the right side of the heart, ventricles on the left side of the heart.

12.28 Ebstein's anomaly is a congenital malformation that is most accurately described as:

A. Inferior displacement of the mitral valve, abnormal closure of the mitral valve on M mode.
B. Superior displacement of the tricuspid valve into atrialized chamber, tricuspid regurgitation, arrhythmias.
C. Inferior displacement of the tricuspid valve, tricuspid regurgitation, arrhythmias, abnormal closure of the tricuspid valve on M mode.
D. Inferior displacement of the tricuspid valve, aortic overriding of the ventricular septum, ventricular septal defect.

12.29 Valvular pulmonic stenosis is characterized on echocardiography by a:

A. High-pitched systolic Doppler flow over 2 m/s.
B. Harsh, turbulent diastolic Doppler jet over 2 m/s.
C. Smooth, uniform waveform on the Doppler tracing measuring at least 100 cm/s.
D. Harsh, turbulent systolic Doppler jet over 2 m/s; the leaflets appear thickened and domed.

12.30 A complete absence of the right ventricular outflow tract and pulmonic valve is representative of:

A. Transposition of the great arteries.
B. Truncus arteriosus.
C. Double-outlet right ventricle.
D. Pulmonary atresia.

12.31 In tricuspid atresia, the systemic venous return must cross which structure to provide blood to the left heart?

    A. Patent foramen ovale.
    B. Secundum atrial septal defect.
    C. Interventricular septal defect.
    D. A and B.

12.32 Which of the following statements are *false* regarding right ventricular volume overload?

Right ventricular volume overload is seen in patients with:

    A. Pulmonary stenosis.
    B. Atrial septal defects.
    C. Tetralogy of Fallot.
    D. Subpulmonary stenosis.
    E. A and D.

12.33 On the parasternal long-axis view, a dilated circular structure behind the left atrium most likely represents:

    A. The descending aorta.
    B. Pulmonary venous return.
    C. Persistent left superior vena cava.
    D. A coronary sinus.

12.34 A linear echo band seen within the left atrium from the atrial septum to the lateral wall may be representative of:

    A. A false tendon.
    B. Cor triatriatum.
    C. Chordae tendinese.
    D. Flail mitral leaflet.

12.35 In patients with an endocardial cushion defect, the cardiac lesions one should look for include:

    A. Cleft mitral valve, atrioventricular regurgitation, primum atrial septal defect, ventricular septal defect.

    B. Cleft mitral valve, patent foramen ovale cordis, membranous septal defect.

    C. Abnormal tricuspid valve, pulmonary stenosis, atrial septal defect.

    D. Abnormal atrioventricular valves with regurgitation, right ventricular volume overload, left ventricular hypertrophy.

12.36 A condition in which valvular chordal attachments adhere to both sides of the ventricular septum is known as:

    A. Valvular atresia.

    B. Ventricular septal defect with tricuspid atresia.

    C. Straddling atrioventricular valves.

    D. Ebstein's anomaly.

12.37 In aortic atresia, echocardiographic findings are:

    A. Normal left ventricular size and function, bicuspid aortic valve, supravalvular aortic stenosis.

    B. Hyperplasia of the left ventricle, atretic distal aorta, bicuspid aortic valve.

    C. Hyperplastic left ventricle, abnormal mitral valve.

    D. Hypoplasia of the left ventricle, atretic proximal aorta, aortic stenosis.

12.38 In patients with infundibular pulmonic stenosis, the Doppler tracing would show increased velocity caused by:

    A. Hypertrophy of the muscle bands in the inflow portion of the right ventricle.

    B. Hypertrophy of the pulmonic annulus.

    C. Hypertrophied muscle bands in the outflow portion of the right ventricle.

    D. Hypertrophy of the valvular tissue in the pulmonary artery.

12.39 A condition in which the left ventricular papillary muscles are closer than normal or fused to form a single papillary muscle is:

    A. Unifocal papillary muscle anomaly.
    B. Unicuspid mitral valve.
    C. Hypertrophied mitral valve.
    D. Parachute mitral valve.

PART II

THE PHYSICS
OF ULTRASOUND

THIRTEEN

PHYSICAL PRINCIPLES AND INSTRUMENTATION

13.0 The term *frequency* is defined by:

    A. The media through which sound travels.
    B. Propagation speed of sound through tissue.
    C. The source of a sound.
    D. The boundary layer.
    E. Reflection and refraction.

Sound waves are described by the following terms: (True or False)

    13.1 Frequency.
    13.2 Amplitude.
    13.3 Perpendicular incidence.
    13.4 Band width.
    13.5 Propagation speed.

13.6 The term for the output of batteries is:

    A. Direct current.
    B. Indirect current.
    C. Direct frequency.
    D. Alternating frequency.
    E. Alternating current.

13.7 Household alternating current generally has a frequency of:

    A. .20 Hertz.
    B. .60 Hertz.
    C. 110 Hertz.
    D. 220 Hertz.
    E. 400 Hertz.

13.8 Propagation speed is dependent upon:

    A. The source of the sound wave.
    B. The amplitude of the sound wave.
    C. The wavelength.
    D. The medium through which the sound wave passes.
    E. The intensity of the sound wave.

13.9 Ultrasound waves do *not* include which of the following characteristics:

    A. Rarefaction.
    B. Pressure.
    C. Particle motion.
    D. Density.
    E. Temperature.

13.10 As the frequency of an acoustic variable increases, the wavelength:

    A. Decreases.
    B. Increases.
    C. Stays the same.
    D. Is unaffected.

13.11 The term *period* is related to frequency because it is:

    A. Equal to frequency.
    B. Increases as frequency increases.
    C. One-tenth of frequency.
    D. The reciprocal of frequency.
    E. Three times wavelength.

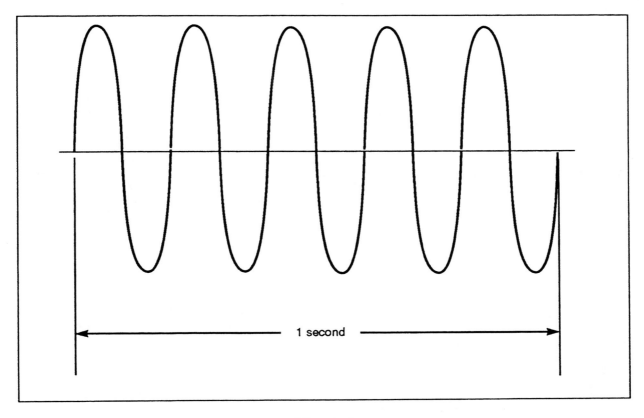

Figure 4

13.12 In Figure 4, what is the frequency?

    A. 10 Hertz.
    B.   7 Hertz.
    C.   5 Hertz.
    D. 2.5 Hertz.
    E. 16 Hertz.

13.13 What is the period of the above frequency?

    A.   .5
    B.   .25
    C. 2.0
    D. .20
    E.   .02

13.14 Intensity is equal to:

    A. Power/area.
    B. Area/power.
    C. Amplitude/distance.
    D. Spatial pulse length/attenuation.

13.15 Ultrasound is defined as a frequency:

    A. Lower than 20 Hz.
    B. Greater than 20 kHz.
    C. Greater than 20 MHz.
    D. Greater than 20 Hz.
    E. Greater than 20 GHz.

Which of the following is/are *true* regarding frequency?

    13.16 It is defined as the number of complete cycles per unit of time.
    13.17 1 cycle per second equals 1 hertz.
    13.18 10,000 cycles per second equals 1 megahertz.
    13.19 1000 cycles per second equals 1 kilohertz.

13.20 Power is defined as:

    A. Work/force.
    B. Force/time.
    C. Work/time.
    D. Mass/acceleration.
    E. Force/work.

13.21 Power divided by the beam area is equal to the:

    A. Probe angle.
    B. Speed of ultrasound.
    C. Velocity of blood.
    D. Intensity.
    E. Attenuation.

13.22 Units of acoustic power output are:

    A. W/cm^2.
    B. N/s^2.
    C. dB/cm.
    D. MHz/cm.
    E. V/cm^2.

13.23 The strength of a sound beam is best described by which two parameters?

    A. Amplitude and frequency.
    B. Amplitude and wavelength.
    C. Amplitude and intensity.
    D. Intensity and frequency.
    E. Frequency and wavelength.

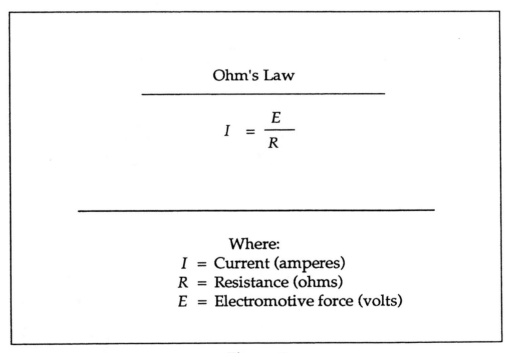

Figure 5

Using Ohm's law as shown in Figure 5, solve the following equations.

13.24 $E = 4$, $R = 2$, $I = ?$

    A. 4
    B. 2
    C. 1
    D. 4.2
    E. 8

13.25 $I = 12$, $R = 3$, $E = ?$

    A. 16
    B. 4
    C. 2.5
    D. 36
    E. 12

13.26 $I = 28$, $E = 56$, $R = ?$

    A. 82
    B. 15
    C. 2
    D. 4
    E. 6

Using the following analogy to Ohm's law, answer the questions below:

$$P_2 = P_1 - (Q \times R_{seg})$$

13.27 As the flow (Q) increases P_2 does which of the following?

    A. Increases.
    B. Decreases.
    C. Remains the same.
    D. Increases to the fourth power.
    E. Decreases to the fourth power.

13.28 Using the equation in Figure 6, what happens when R_{seg} increases?

    A. P_1 Increases.
    B. P_2 Increases.
    C. P_1 decreases.
    D. P_2 decreases.
    E. R_{seg} decreases.

13.29 If P_1 increases, P_2 does which of the following?

    A. Increases.
    B. Decreases.
    C. Does not change.
    D. Becomes a function of R_{seg}.
    E. Falls to the fourth power.

13.30 If $P_1 = 100$, $Q = 12$, and $R_{seg} = 3$, what is P_2?

    A. 46
    B. 32
    C. 36
    D. 64
    E. 33

13.31 If $P_2 = 120$, $Q = 6$ and $R_{seg} = 5$, what is P_1?

    A. 200
    B. 150
    C. 140
    D. 130
    E. 120

13.32 Resistance to flow is governed by viscosity, length of a segment or segments, and the radius of the segment. If the radius of a vessel segment is decreased by 50%, what does the resistance do?

    A. Increases by 2 times.
    B. Increases by 4 times.
    C. Increases by 16 times.
    D. Decreases by 2 times.
    E. Remains the same.

13.33 Hydrostatic pressure is defined as:

    A. The gravitational pressure from the head to the feet.
    B. The dynamic pressure minus the gravitational pressure.
    C. The intracardiac (left ventricle) pressure.
    D. The dynamic pressure minus the weight of the blood.
    E. Equal to the weight of a column of blood extending from the heart to the level of pressure measurement.

13.34 The cosine of 90° is:

    A. 0.0000
    B. 0.4545
    C. 0.5000
    D. 0.7070
    E. 1.0000

FOURTEEN

PROPAGATION SPEED

14.0 The propagation speed of sound is determined by:

    A. The frequency of the sound wave.
    B. The intensity of the sound wave.
    C. Attenuation of the sound wave.
    D. Reflection of the sound wave.
    E. The medium through which the sound wave passes.

14.1 If the stiffness of a material increases, the propagation speed of a wave passing through it:

    A. Decreases.
    B. Increases.
    C. Stays the same.
    D. Doubles.

14.2 Wavelength is measured in:

    A. Hertz.
    B. Microseconds.
    C. Millimeters.
    D. Impedance.
    E. Rayls.

14.3 The units of attenuation are:

    A. Frequencies.
    B. Decibels.
    C. Milliseconds.
    D. Rayls.
    E. Centimeters per second.

14.4 As frequency increases, the attenuation coefficient:

    A. Decreases.
    B. Increases.
    C. Stays the same.
    D. Scatters.

14.5 The propagation speed of sound through soft tissue is:

    A. 1450 m/s.
    B. 8000 m/s.
    C. 1540 m/s.
    D. 5000 m/s.
    E. 1230 m/s.

14.6 The propagation speed of sound is similar in all of the following examples *except*:

    A. The liver.
    B. Fat.
    C. Muscle.
    D. Bone.
    E. Subcutaneous tissue.

14.7 Reduction in the strength of a sound beam as it travels through a medium is defined as:

    A. Wavelength.
    B. Attenuation.
    C. Propagation speed.
    D. Frequency.
    E. Constant shift.

14.8 Attenuation of a sound beam through tissue occurs because of the following reasons *except*:

    A. Uniform tissue density.
    B. Reflection of sound waves.
    C. Scattering of sound waves.
    D. Absorption of ultrasonic energy.
    E. Depth of sound penetration.

14.9 The estimated absorption or attenuation of ultrasound in soft tissue is:

    A. 10 dB/cm/MHz.
    B. 20 dB/cm/MHz.
    C. 1 dB/cm/MHz.
    D. 2 dB/cm/MHz.
    E. 16 dB/cm/MHz.

14.10 The absorption, reflection, and scattering of a sound beam can be described best as:

    A. Frequency.
    B. Propagation speed.
    C. Wavelength.
    D. Attenuation.
    E. Intensity.

14.11 The depth of penetration of ultrasound in tissue can be determined roughly by the formula for attenuation: 1 dB/cm/MHz. Simply stated, this relationship implies that for each million cycles per second ultrasound frequency used, the signal will be attenuated approximately 1 decibel for every centimeter of tissue it must pass through. Which of the following statements can be inferred from this relationship?

    A. The lower the transmitted frequency, the lower the effective signal penetration.
    B. The higher the transmitted frequency, the lower the subsequent tissue penetration.
    C. The higher the pulse repetition frequency (PRF), the greater the subsequent tissue penetration.
    D. The broader the dynamic range, the greater the subsequent tissue penetration.

14.12 Which one of the following best describes the clinical application of the concept "dynamic range?"

    A. The ability to provide high resolution at extreme tissue depths.
    B. The ability to differentiate structures of slightly different acoustic impedances.
    C. The ability to image the vessel dynamics as they occur within the body.
    D. The concept of providing dynamic vessel information and Doppler flow information in a single system.

14.13 Dynamic range is absolutely limited by:

    A. The fact that ultrasound travels through different tissue layers at slightly different propagation speeds.
    B. The use of analog versus digital scan converter technology within the imaging system.
    C. The fact that calcium reflects virtually all ultrasound that strikes it.
    D. The fact that cathode ray tubes used in image display have a fixed display dynamic range of 36 dB.

FIFTEEN

THE ULTRASOUND TRANSDUCER

15.0 Spatial pulse length is equal to:

    A. The wavelength times the number of cycles in the pulse.
    B. The wavelength minus the number of cycles in the pulse.
    C. The wavelength times axial resolution.
    D. The wavelength times .05
    E. The period times pulse duration.
    F. Pulse repetition.

15.1 An ultrasound probe with a frequency of 10 MHz will have a period of:

    A. 1.00 microseconds.
    B. 1.00 seconds.
    C. 0.13 microseconds.
    D. 0.20 microseconds.
    E. 0.10 microseconds.

15.2 Wavelength is equal to the propagation speed:

    A. Times frequency.
    B. Divided by frequency.
    C. Times density.
    D. Divided by period.
    E. Times pulse repetition frequency.

15.3 Spatial pulse length is equal to the number of cycles in the pulse:

    A. Divided by wavelength.
    B. Divided by frequency.
    C. Times frequency.
    D. Times wavelength.
    E. Times 1.54.

15.4 In ultrasound imaging, resolution is described as:

    A. Axial and lateral.
    B. Proximal and distal.
    C. Band width and half intensity depth.
    D. Lateral and transverse.
    E. Spatial pulse length and axial.

15.5 As frequency increases, axial resolution:

    A. Is reduced.
    B. Stays the same.
    C. Improves.
    D. Is dampened.
    E. Affects the near zone length.

15.6 Axial resolution is described in:

    A. Milliseconds.
    B. Centimeters.
    C. Decibels.
    D. Millivolts.
    E. Millimeters.

15.7 In a Doppler transducer, piezoelectric crystals provide all of the following activities, *except*:

    A. Generation and detection of sound waves.
    B. Conversion of pressure into electrical signals.
    C. Conversion of electrical signals into mechanical vibrations.
    D. Conversion of mechanical vibrations into electrical signals.
    E. Conversion of pressure into mechanical vibrations.

15.8 In a continuous-wave Doppler, the area where the transmitting and receiving beam profiles cross paths is known as the:

    A. Zone of sensitivity.
    B. Sample volume.
    C. Area of detection.
    D. Transition point.
    E. Far field.

15.9 The frequency of a transducer is determined by:

    A. The number of times the crystal is electronically stimulated.
    B. The mechanical properties and shape of the crystal.
    C. The band width of the transducer.
    D. The size and shape of the transducer.
    E. A and D.

15.10 Focusing a sound beam with its power remaining constant:

    A. Decreases intensity at the focal point.
    B. Increases intensity at the focal point.
    C. Causes no change in intensity at the focal point.
    D. Decreases wavelength.
    E. Increases wavelength.

15.11 Which of the following transducer arrays is *not* indicative of a mechanical real-time system configuration?

    A. A single transducer that is reciprocated in a given arc.
    B. A single transducer reflected off a reciprocating acoustical mirror.
    C. Multiple piezoelectric elements that are positioned like blades of a fan, electronically timed to fire at a preselected window.
    D. Multiple piezoelectric elements, positioned side to side, electronically stimulated to operate in sequence.

In cardiac imaging axial resolution is the determinant that: (True or False)

15.12 Differentiates soft plaque from blood.
15.13 Resolves two targets positioned perpendicular to each other within the plane of beam propagation.
15.14 Improves the observer's ability to estimate wall thickness.
15.15 Determines the absolute depth of penetration of the ultrasound beam at a given frequency.

15.16 Axial resolution is determined chiefly by:

    A. Beam width.
    B. Transducer diameter.
    C. Transducer frequency and spatial pulse length.
    D. Half-amplitude frequency.

Lateral resolution is determined by: (True or False)

15.17 Transducer frequency.
15.18 Transducer (*f#*) focal length.
15.19 Spatial pulse length.
15.20 Pulse repetition frequency.
15.21 Half-amplitude frequency.

15.22 Determinants of resolution in two-dimensional space are:

    A. Axial and logarithmic.
    B. Axial and radial.
    C. Axial and lateral.
    D. Sagittal and transverse.

SIXTEEN

PULSE-ECHO IMAGING

16.0 Which ONE of the following statements most accurately describes M-mode methods of echo display?

    A. Dynamic plaque characteristics can be related to known disease states, as in analysis of abnormal cardiac function.

    B. Extended dynamic range capability is made possible by compression of multiple image vectors into a single column.

    C. Motion patterns of the vessel walls can be studied, but display of local vessel abnormalities is of limited usefulness.

    D. The presence of fresh thrombus can be detected most reliably with this method in most patients.

Which of the following statements is True/False regarding amplitude-mode (A-mode) echo display?

    16.1 Differentiation of echo intensity is related by relative height of the displayed echo pattern.

    16.2 Plaque contour can be readily assessed.

    16.3 Differentiation of artifact echoes from reflections from true anatomic structures is simple.

    16.4 It is the only method of ultrasound transmission that can penetrate the skull, allowing for determination of midline brain shifts.

16.5 Dynamic range is:

    A. The upper limit of Doppler signal detection sensitivity, beyond which aliasing occurs.

    B. The real-time motion analysis of the vessel made possible by high-speed computer processing.

    C. The range of displayed gray scale between the lowest- and highest-magnitude signals the system can detect.

    D. An advanced, infinitely variable depth gain compensation process.

16.6 A given imaging system's dynamic range capability would largely determine:

    A. Plaque contour irregularities.

    B. Tandem lesions.

    C. Subtle acoustical changes within a plaque.

    D. Tortuosity.

16.7 Dynamic range is measured in:

    A. Centimeters per second.

    B. Millimeters.

    C. Decibels.

    D. Any of these, depending on the specific instrumentation used.

16.8 B-scan instrumentation differs from B-mode real-time instrumentation in that:

    A. B-scan images, when displayed in compound fashion, can render three-dimensional views of the carotid vasculature.

    B. Essentially no difference exists between the two technologies, since rapid hand-manipulated movement of the B-scan transducer can approximate the same frame rates as obtained with real-time B mode .

    C. B-mode real-time instrumentation is so named to denote the use of high speed computers that can acquire and display information more rapidly than conventional B-scan techniques.

    D. B-mode real-time instrumentation is comparatively limited in its ability to display broad dynamic range and discrete resolution owing to the effects of signal digitization often used in the instrumentation.

16.9 B-mode imaging provides information on:

    A. Lateral position.
    B. Depth.
    C. Echo amplitude.
    D. All of these.

Acoustical information is converted into image data through use of: (True or False)

    16.10 Analog scan converter circuitry.
    16.11 Fast Fourier transform analysis of the reflected ultrasound spectra.
    16.12 Phase/cycle shift detection circuitry.
    16.13 Digital scan converter circuitry.

Which of the following is/are true when describing the principal benefits of digital scan conversion? (True or False)

    16.14 Computer circuitry can acquire and display information at different rates of time.
    16.15 An infinitely variable gray-scale range is obtainable (within the limits of video display technology).
    16.16 Image-processing capabilities such as digital subtraction and enhancement techniques can be employed.
    16.17 Increased signal penetration is made possible by digital scan conversion.

16.18 The principal benefit of analog scan conversion is that:

    A. Computer circuitry can acquire and display information at different rates of time.
    B. An infinitely variable gray scale range is obtainable (within the limits of video display technology).
    C. Image-processing capabilities such as digital subtraction and enhancement techniques can be employed.
    D. Increased signal penetration is made possible.

SEVENTEEN

DOPPLER ULTRASOUND

17.0 The term *Doppler signal processing* describes the:

  A. Doppler shift.
  B. Reflected frequency.
  C. Comparison of the reflected frequency and the transmitting frequency.
  D. Transmitting frequency.
  E. Oscillator frequency.

17.1 In Doppler ultrasound, the blood acts mainly as:

  A. An ultrasonic field.
  B. A small reflector.
  C. An absorbent field.
  D. A sound source.
  E. An attenuator.

17.2 Which of the following Doppler frequencies would result in the shallowest penetration depth?

  A.   2 MHz.
  B. 20 MHz.
  C.   8 MHz.
  D. 10 MHz.
  E.   4 MHz.

17.3 "Ultrasound backscattered from moving blood is shifted in frequency by an amount proportional to the blood velocity." The statement describes:

    A. The reflected beam.
    B. Movement of the reflector.
    C. Movement in the ultrasound field.
    D. The Doppler shift.
    E. Attenuation.

17.4 The reflected Doppler signal contains how many frequencies?

    A. Only one.
    B. It depends on the probe frequency.
    C. It is proportional to the blood-cell velocities.
    D. No one knows.
    E. One hundred.

17.5 The frequency of ultrasound is determined by the number of oscillations per second produced by:

    A. An oscillator.
    B. The particles of the medium that it is propagating.
    C. Band width and intensity.
    D. Scattering.
    E. Electronic propagation.

17.6 When an ultrasound reflector is moving away from a source, the reflected frequency may be:

    A. Twice the incident frequency.
    B. Three times the incident frequency.
    C. Equal to the incident frequency.
    D. The incident frequency times 1.25.
    E. One-half the incident frequency.

17.7 The largest Doppler shift occurs when the beam of ultrasound insonates the vessel at a:

    A. 90 degree angle.
    B. 45 degree angle.
    C. 0 degree angle.
    D. 30 degree angle.
    E. 15 degree angle.

17.8 Movement toward a transducer produces an upward shift in the reflected frequency. Circuits within a directional Doppler would detect this as:

    A. Continuous flow.
    B. Antegrade flow.
    C. Pulsed flow.
    D. Retrograde flow.
    E. Pulsatile flow.

17.9 The one factor in the Doppler equation that is unknown when using Doppler ultrasound by itself is:

    A. The angle of incidence.
    B. The transmitting frequency.
    C. The change in frequency (delta f).
    D. The speed of sound in soft tissue.
    E. The velocity shift of red blood cells.

17.10 A pulse repetition frequency (PRF) less than twice Doppler shift frequency will result in:

    A. Cavitation.
    B. Aliasing.
    C. Increased intensity.
    D. Decreased intensity.
    E. Increased attenuation.

17.11 The Doppler frequency shift heard on a speaker or seen on a spectrum analyzer is the difference between the transmitted frequency and the:

    A. Doppler probe frequency.
    B. Received frequency.
    C. Transmitted intensity.
    D. Speed of sound through tissue.
    E. Angle of incidence.

17.12 Although continuous-wave Doppler instruments are less complex, only pulsed Doppler allows for:

    A. Depth location.
    B. Frequency shift.
    C. Blood flow determination.
    D. Spectrum analysis.
    E. Directional separation.

17.13 Which of the following artifacts *cannot* be detected while using full spectral analysis?

    A. Significant background noise.
    B. High-amplitude, low-frequency signal from arterial wall movement.
    C. Probe frequency inadequate to fully insonate the vessel.
    D. Signals recorded simultaneously from two or more vessels.

When a pulsed Doppler is used, which characteristics are used in determining the shape and size of the sample volume? (True or False)

    17.14 The transmitted pulse length.
    17.15 The beam width.
    17.16 The acoustic interface.
    17.17 The gated range width.
    17.18 The analog output characteristics.

17.19 Determination of the mean frequency and the conversion of the Doppler signal into an analog signal are usually performed by a:

    A. Unidirectional Doppler.
    B. Bidirectional Doppler.
    C. Zero-crossing detector.
    D. Fast Fourier transformer.

17.20 Spectral analysis is often referred to as a process of:

    A. Separating a signal into electrical components that define the greatest velocity flow.
    B. Combining all frequencies received from a Doppler signal and rearranging them to allow maximum display of the flow velocities.
    C. Separating a signal into its individual frequency components so that each component is relative to the original frequency shifts when visualized.
    D. Separating a signal into different frequency components so that the intensity of each signal can be visualized.

17.21 Spectral analysis displays, as components of the Doppler signal, the:

    A. Amplitude, frequency, capacitance.
    B. Capacitance, time, frequency.
    C. Time, amplitude, voltage.
    D. Voltage, capacitance, frequency.
    E. Amplitude, time, frequency.

17.22 Frequencies displayed by Doppler spectral analysis depend on:

    A. Simple waveforms.
    B. Flow characteristics.
    C. Average velocities.
    D. Percentage of change.
    E. Average amplitudes.

17.23 The fast Fourier transform allows the technologist to:

    A. Analyze a plethysmographic signal.
    B. Display the velocity distributions.
    C. Display a real-time analysis of Doppler spectra.
    D. Convert a Doppler signal into an analog waveform.
    E. B and C.

17.24 A unique advantage of fast Fourier transform (FFT) spectral analysis over zero-crossing analog analysis is that:

   A. FFT analysis avoids the problems of aliasing common in analog detection systems.
   B. FFT extracts and displays the separate component frequencies of the Doppler flow velocity shift.
   C. Calculation of flow velocity can be determined only by using FFT analysis.
   D. FFT spectral analysis cannot calculate flow acceleration at low frequency shift values; it offers no clinical advantage.

17.25 Of the following statements the one that is *true* regarding fast Fourier transform spectral analysis is that:

   A. It is used to analyze the individual frequency components of a composite Doppler frequency-shift spectrum.
   B. It is responsible for the phenomenon of signal aliasing in extreme frequency-shift states.
   C. Simultaneous, separate display of forward and reverse flow components can confuse the system, rendering a frequency-shift pattern that is artificially blunted.
   D. It is accurate only when used in conjunction with continuous-wave or pulsed Doppler systems using a large sample volume gate.

Which of the following statements is/are True/False regarding the difference between pulsed and continuous-wave Doppler:

   17.26 Pulsed Doppler operates at a lower transmitting power owing to its intermittent operation and is therefore clinically safer than continuous-wave Doppler.
   17.27 Continuous-wave Doppler can penetrate bone and is therefore the system of choice in mapping the second portion of the vertebral artery.
   17.28 Continuous-wave Doppler systems cannot alias, in spite of accelerated flow velocity states.
   17.29 Flow velocity data can be determined only from continuous-wave Doppler.

Which of the following is/are True/False regarding continuous-wave Doppler?

17.30 Signals from different depths cannot be differentiated.
17.31 Vessels that lie above or below the overlapped transducer-reception paths cannot be studied.
17.32 The two transducer elements are always in operation.
17.33 Aliasing can occur at frequency shifts above a range specific to the instrumentation used.

The following questions are based on the Doppler flow velocity equation:

$$\Delta F = \frac{2FV \, (\cos \phi)}{C}$$

Figure 7

17.34 In this equation the audible Doppler signal is the result of:

A. Frequency changes in the reflected ultrasound beam produced by acoustical impedance changes at different tissue layers.
B. Frequency changes in the reflected ultrasound beam produced by stenosis within the vessel.
C. Frequency changes in the reflected ultrasound beam produced by movement of the red blood cells through the vessel.
D. Algorithms derived by computer on the basis of time/depth processing of the reflected ultrasound beam.

17.35 Which of the following would produce a Doppler frequency shift?

A. Movement of the probe on the skin above the area being studied.
B. Wall motion.
C. Movement of a valve or thrombus within the heart.
D. All of the above.

The absolute maximum pitch of the reflected Doppler signal may be influenced by: (True or False)

17.36 The designated transducer frequency.

17.37 The angulation of the ultrasound beam with respect to the movement path of the target studied.

17.38 The direction of travel of the target with respect to the ultrasound transducer.

17.39 The velocity of the moving target.

17.40 Duplex ultrasound imaging systems:

A. May use only continuous-wave Doppler because of the extremely high flow-velocity states that may exist in a diseased carotid vessel.

B. May use pulsed Doppler because of the need to stage image and Doppler-transducer operation sequentially so that accurate sample gate placement may be achieved.

C. Cannot use continuous-wave or pulsed Doppler with analog signal analysis circuitry because of interference from the reflected imaging signal.

D. None of these.

17.41 Aliasing is :

A. The act of registering at a hotel under an assumed name.

B. The erroneous presentation of Doppler flow data.

C. The waveform display seen when the Doppler gain is overdriven.

D. The waveform display seen when the continuous-wave Doppler beam overlaps an artery and a vein.

E. Using an incorrectly sized Doppler.

17.42 Aliasing can occur:

A. Only in pulsed Doppler systems.

B. In either pulsed or continuous-wave Doppler systems.

C. Only in continuous-wave Doppler systems.

D. Only in duplex imaging systems.

17.43 The pulse repetition frequency (PRF) is described as:

    A. The transmitted frequency of the Doppler ultrasound beam.
    B. The rate at which the continuous-wave Doppler ultrasound transducer is stimulated.
    C. The speed at which the sound pulse travels through a given tissue structure.
    D. The rate at which the pulsed Doppler transducer is stimulated.

17.44 Aliasing will occur with frequency shifts at a level:

    A. Equal to that of the system's pulse repetition frequency.
    B. Equal to 60% of the system's pulse repetition frequency.
    C. Equal to 50% of the system's pulse repetition frequency.
    D. Equal to two times the system's pulse repetition frequency.

17.45 Aliasing does *not* occur in continuous-wave (CW) Doppler systems because:

    A. Of the higher designated frequencies that can be used with a continuous-wave Doppler.
    B. The transducer is constantly transmitting ultrasound which faithfully recreates the constantly changing flow velocity patterns within the vessel.
    C. Of the inherently greater frequency shift produced by the relatively stronger broadcast signal.
    D. The sampling of the entire vessel averages the flow velocities to minimize the peak systolic velocity and more faithfully reproduces the true flow velocity patterns in the vessel.

If a pulsed Doppler transducer of 5 MHz is used with a pulse repetition frequency (PRF) of 15 kHz, which of the following frequency shifts would produce aliasing? (True or False)

    17.46 5 kHz.
    17.47 6.25 kHz.
    17.48 8 kHz.
    17.49 30 kHz.

To minimize aliasing in a given situation, the technologist would attempt the following: (True or False)

17.50 Increasing the transmitting power of the Doppler.

17.51 Switching to continuous-wave Doppler.

17.52 Attempting to achieve an angle of incidence that minimizes the maximum detected frequency shift.

17.53 There is nothing the operator can do to minimize the potential for aliasing.

17.54 Fast Fourier transform (FFT) spectrum analysis derives what part(s) of the following data from the Doppler signal?

A. Peak frequency.
B. Spectral band width.
C. Phase shift.
D. All of the above.

17.55 The Doppler signal may be analyzed by means of:

A. The single time interval power/frequency display.
B. The real-time gray scale histogram display.
C. The pie graph display.
D. Any of the above; the numeric data are not altered by the means of statistical display.

17.56 When spectral analysis is used with a continuous-wave Doppler, which differences would one expect in comparison to pulsed Doppler recordings of the same vessel?

A. Higher peak velocity.
B. Increased windowing.
C. Reduced windowing.
D. Lower peak velocity.
E. No difference at all.

17.57 All of the following must be known to calculate the velocity by the Doppler technique *except*:

    A. The beam/vessel angle of incidence.
    B. The emitting frequency of ultrasound.
    C. The shifted frequency of the returning ultrasound.
    D. The carotid blood flow.
    E. The speed of ultrasound in tissue.

17.58 Simultaneously, two pure musical notes are played constantly, one at 60 Hz, the other at 80 Hz. Which statement describes the presentation of these on a time-domain spectrum analyzer?

    A. One straight line at 140 Hz.
    B. One sine wave centered at 140 Hz.
    C. Two straight lines, one at 60 Hz, one at 80 Hz.
    D. Two sine waves, one centered at 60 Hz, one centered at 80 Hz.
    E. One sine wave centered at 70 Hz.

Using the Doppler shift equation for velocity, solve the following:

17.59

$$\text{delta } F = 4.6 \text{ kHz}$$
$$F = 2 \text{ MHz}$$
$$\text{Cos } \varnothing = 45°$$

    A. 2.53 m/s.
    B. 25.3 m/s.
    C. .253 m/s.
    D. .0253 m/s.

17.60

$$\text{delta } F = 6.8 \text{ kHz}$$
$$F = 3 \text{ MHz}$$
$$\text{Cos } \varnothing = 45°$$

    A. 2.53 m/s.
    B. 2.49 m/s.
    C. 24.9 m/s.
    D. 2.49 m/s.
    E. 25.3 m/s.

17.61

delta F = 12.2 kHz
F = 2500 MHz
Cos ø = 45°

A. 14.06 m/s.
B.   9.12 m/s.
C.   7.08 m/s.
D.   4.69 m/s.
E.   5.36 m/s.

17.62

delta F = 4.6 kHz
F = 3 MHz
Cos ø = 0°

A. 2.53 m/s.
B. 1.31 m/s.
C. 2.34 m/s.
D. 1.36 m/s.
E. 2.36 m/s.

17.63 Finding in a patient are a maximum delta F of 6.7 kHz, an F of 3 MHz, and a cosine ø of 0° at the aortic valve. The peak gradient across the valve is:

A. 14.59.
B. 19.13.
C.   1.91.
D. 15.2.

17.64 An aortic valve has a delta F of 10 kHz, an F of 2000 kHz, and a cosine ø of 0.70. What is the pressure gradient?

A. 121 m/s.
B. 121 mmHg.
C. 1.21 m/s.
D. 12.1 mmHg.
E. .121 mmHg.

EIGHTEEN

IMAGE FEATURES AND ARTIFACTS

18.0 The physical phenomenon of refraction is:

 A. The concept of bending of the ultrasound beam at tissue interfaces.
 B. The concept of spatial pulse length affecting axial resolution.
 C. The brightest signal that can be displayed on a standard cathode ray monitor.
 D. The lateral resolution and pulse length.

18.1 Reverberation or "ring-down" artifact is often seen from the walls nearest the imaging transducer. This same phenomenon is not seen in the other walls (more distant from the transducer) because:

 A. The acoustical mismatch between tissue and blood is much greater than the acoustical mismatch of blood and tissue.
 B. The spatial pulse length used in most instrumentation is so short that ricocheting of the ultrasound signal occurs only in the tissue edge nearest the probe; the signal is too weak at greater depths to produce this phenomenon.
 C. Reverberation artifact is a function of beam width; therefore this phenomenon does not occur in systems using a comparatively narrow beam width.
 D. Reverberation does occur in the more distant walls and is obscured by reflections from anatomically adjacent tissue.

18.2 Bony structures and calcification often produce acoustical shadowing because:

    A. Calcified structures have a high coefficient of absorption so that they soak up ultrasound energy.

    B. Calcified structures have a high refractory coefficient and bend the ultrasound beam to such an extent that the returning ultrasound energy is directed away from the receiving transducer.

    C. Calcified structures allow for initial penetration of the ultrasound beam, but the resultant ultrasound energy is locked into the structure as a diminishing series of low-amplitude reverberations.

    D. Calcified structures possess a high reflective coefficient and absorb the minute fraction of ultrasound energy that can penetrate them.

18.3 The following contribute(s) to the inherently low Doppler signal-to-noise ratio:

    A. The transmitted power.

    B. The angle of Doppler-beam incidence (with respect to the blood-flow path).

    C. The strong reflection coefficient of red blood cells to ultrasound.

    D. The poor reflection coefficient of red blood cells to ultrasound.

    E. A and C.

NINETEEN

QUALITY ASSURANCE

The performance rating of imaging systems is determined by : (True or False)

19.0 Axial resolution.
19.1 Range accuracy.
19.2 Registration accuracy.
19.3 Acoustic output.
19.4 Gray-scale dynamic range.

19.5 The measurement of relative system sensitivity is obtained by:

A. Setting range low and having high compensation.
B. Setting gain or attenuation high and using no compensation.
C. Setting gain low and having no compensation.
D. Setting range high and having low compensation.

Axial resolution measured with the AIUM test object shows: (True or False)

19.6 A reflection of the best possible axial resolution of the imaging instrument.
19.7 A reflection of a fairly accurate resolution compared to the actual resolution of the instrument.
19.8 Separations of from 3 to 6 mm.
19.9 Separations of from 1 to 5 mm.
19.10 Depth of the rods designated as rod group scanned from face A.

19.11 Gray-scale dynamic range is:

    A. The difference between the gain or attenuation settings (dB) that produce (1) barely discernible and (2) maximally deflected displays for the same reflection.

    B. The closeness of the gain or attenuation (dB) that produces (1) discernible and maximum deflection of displays (A, B, or M mode for the same reflection).

    C. A function of the lateral resolution plus the axial resolution.

    D. The ability of imaging systems to compensate for inaccuracies in depth or range resolution.

19.12 Joules/cm^2 is an expression of:

    A. Time and area.

    B. Distance and area.

    C. Intensity and area.

    D. Voltage and area.

    E. Heat and area.

19.13 In pulsed ultrasound systems, the operating frequency is determined by the:

    A. Tissue.

    B. Pulses.

    C. Transducer.

    D. Memory.

    E. Display.

TWENTY

BIOLOGIC EFFECTS

20.0 According to the biologic effects committee of AIUM as of October 1982, "No independently confirmed significant bioeffects in mammalian tissues have been reported at intensities below . . .":

    A. 1 W/cm^2.
    B. 10 W/cm^2.
    C. 100 mW/cm^2.
    D. 500 mW/cm^2.
    E. 1000 mW/cm^2.

20.1 Two bioeffects in ultrasound are:

    A. Heat and cavitation.
    B. Vibration and cooling.
    C. Cavitation and cooling.
    D. Intensity and vibration.
    E. Heat and disruption of the cell wall.

20.2 The AIUM statement on in vivo ultrasonic biologic effects states that in ultrasound exposure times of less than 500 seconds and greater than 1 second, such effects have not been demonstrated even at higher intensities, when the product of intensity and exposure time is:

    A. More than 50 joules/cm² and less than 100 joules/cm².
    B. Less than 50 joules/cm².
    C. Less than 25 joules/cm².
    D. Less than 50 mw/cm².
    E. Less than 150 joules/cm².

PART III

ANSWERS

ONE

1.0 **D** In 1978 the American Society of Echocardiography recommended that all echo measurements be taken from the leading edge of each structure so that all laboratories would be using a consistent method. (Guidelines of the American Society of Echocardiography)

1.1 **C** The basilar area of the heart is at a level near the AV valves. (Gardin and Talano)

1.2 **B** The infundibulum is a funnel-shaped passage leading directly out of the right ventricle. (Hagan-8)

1.3 **B** The right subclavian artery arises from the innominate (brachiocephalic trunk). Obviously this answer assumes normal anatomy. (See any general anatomy text)

1.4 **B** (See any general anatomy text)

1.5 **A** The three sections of the arterial wall are the intima, media, and the adventitia. (See any general anatomy text)

1.6 **C** Often people with dextracardia have all organs reversed. (Chung-18)

1.7 **D** *Semilunar* refers to the crescent or half-moon shape of the aortic and pulmonic valves. (Hagan-4)

1.8 **D** The aortic and the pulmonary arteries are described as the great vessels. The aorta delivers oxgenated blood to the body, and the pulmonary artery delivers unoxygenated blood to the lungs. (See any cardiology text)

1.9 **D, E, F, A, C** Note that the **B** notch is seen only when there is interruption in the closure of the mitral valve. (See any basic echocardiography reference)

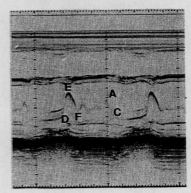

1.10   **A** Anterior right ventricular wall, **B** interventricular septum, and **C** left
ventricular posterior wall. (See any general echocardiography reference)

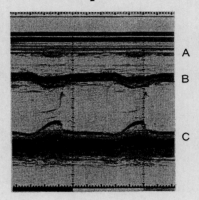

1.11   A. Anterior right ventricular wall
B. Right ventricular outflow tract
C. Anterior aortic wall
D. Aortic valve
E. Posterior aortic wall
F. Left atrium
G. Posterior left atrial wall
(See any basic echocardiography reference)

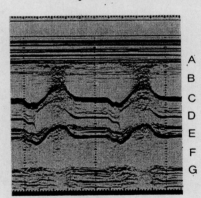

1.12 B   The R wave denotes the electrical stimulation that initiates systole. The Q
wave is not always present and is not an indicator of end systole. Although
the septum is at its maximum posterior motion under normal conditions, it is
susceptible to electrical aberrations and volume and pressure changes and
therefore not consistent for measurement. Only the maximum anterior
motion of the left ventricular posterior wall is consistent for end-systolic
measurement. (Guidelines of the American Society of Echocardiography)

1.13 C At the basal level the M-mode beam is directed through the aorta and left atrium. At the mitral level the septum may still show a pattern consistent with aortic motion. At the apical level the beam would be crossing at an abnormal angle. The midventricular level is most accurate for evaluating septal motion. (Guidelines of the American Society of Echocardiography)

1.14 F The coronary sinus is the terminal portion of the great cardiac vein, and it returns blood to the right atrium. (Weyman-6)

1.15 T A narrow opening on the left coronary cusp of the AV valve at approximately 4 to 5 o'clock may define the ostium (opening) of the left coronary artery. (Hagan-6)

1.16 B The atria and ventricles are always in opposite phases. (See any general cardiology text)

1.17 A The P wave on an ECG is the electrical stimulus that creates the mitral A wave, which coincides with the atrial kick and late diastolic filling. (Feigenbaum-5)

1.18 T

1.19 F

1.20 F

1.21 T

Explanation for 1.18 through 1.21 Early diastolic murmurs are due to aortic or pulmonic insufficiency. (Chung-1)

1.22 A An Austin-Flint murmur is associated with aortic insufficiency. (Weyman-5)

1.23 B Mitral closure normally precedes tricuspid closure by 0.02 to 0.03 second, so that audible splitting (duplication) of the first heart sound is a common and normal occurrence. (Chung-1)

1.24 D Systolic clicks are among the most important physical findings in patients with mitral valve prolapse. The clicks may be single or multiple and may be brought out by changes in position or by using the Valsalva maneuver. (Chung-1)

1.25 D The sounds are sharp and high-pitched. In isolated mitral stenosis, increasing severity of the lesion causes higher atrial pressures and early opening of the valve. A relatively short interval between the aortic component of the second heart sounds and the opening snap (A_2–OS interval) implies severe mitral stenosis. A pericardial knock, which occurs with constrictive pericarditis, is an early diastolic sound that can be confused with an opening snap. (Chung-1)

1.26 T The severity of regurgitation is often inversely related to the duration of the murmur. With severe regurgitation, aortic diastolic pressure falls rapidly and may equalize with ventricular pressure relatively early, causing marked reduction of intensity or cessation of the murmur. Aortic insufficiency may also cause a diastolic rumble at the apex—an Austin-Flint murmur. Pulmonary insufficiency is associated with two forms of murmurs. In pulmonary insufficiency due to pulmonary hypertension, there is a large diastolic gradient. The murmur is high-pitched, follows the second heart sound immediately, and continues throughout diastole. In pulmonary insufficiency caused by valvular disease, there is usually a silent period between the pulmonic second heart sound and the initiation of the murmur, which is relatively low in frequency. (Chung-1)

1.27 F These tumors are located only intracardially.

1.28 T

1.29 F Myxomas can occur in either atrium, on the mitral valve, or in the ventricles.

1.30 T

1.31 T

1.32 F

1.33 T

1.34 F

1.35 T

1.36 F

1.37 T

1.38 T

1.39 B

1.40 T

1.41 B

1.42 D

1.43 T

1.44 T

1.45 T

1.46 T

1.47 T (Chung-1 for 1.30–1.47)

1.48 T All of the diagnostic methods listed should discover dextrocardia. Patients have been known to keep their condition quiet to check your skills. (Chung-1)

1.49 T

1.50 T

1.51 T

1.52 T

Explanation for 1.49 through 1.52 All of the above may be indicators of cardiac disease but are not specifically diagnostic. (Chung-1)

1.53 C Left ventricular stroke volume is directly related to cardiac output. Therefore any decrease in left ventricular stroke volume will reduce cardiac output. Conversely, an increase in left ventricular stroke volume will raise cardiac output. (See any general cardiac Doppler text)

1.54 B Left ventricular contractility will decrease delta P and in doing so will reduce cardiac output. (See any general cardiac Doppler text)

1.55 A A reduction in vessel diameter increases velocity within the constricted segment. A reduction in vessel diameter also increases the likelihood of turbulence, and if the diameter is sufficiently reduced, flow will be reduced (critical stenosis). (See any general cardiac Doppler text)

1.56 A (See any general cardiac Doppler text)

1.57 T Reynold's numbers above 2000 indicate turbulent flow.

1.58 T

1.59 F If any change in pressure occurs, there would be a reduction in pressure/flow.

1.60 T

1.61 T (See any general cardiac Doppler text for 1.57–1.61)

1.62 C See the analogy to Ohm's law. Cardiac output and pressure are governed not by how much blood the heart can put out in a given period but rather by how much blood the peripheral vessels are capable of accepting. With cardiac output halved and peripheral resistance doubled, pressure remains the same.

1.63 C (See any general cardiac Doppler text)

1.64 B

1.65 C

1.66 D

1.67 D (See any general physiology text for 1.64–1.67)

1.68 D The fact that normal blood flow is zero at the vessel wall and highest at center stream is one reason why continuous-wave Dopplers show wider frequency shifts (decreased windowing) when spectrally analyzed. (See any general physiology text)

1.69 C (See any general anatomy text)

1.70 B

1.71 C

1.72 C

1.73 B (See any general physiology text for 1.70–1.73)

TWO

2.0 D Depth control automatically adjusts (or calibrates) depth markers. (Feigenbaum-1)

2.1 F Increasing gain will increase specular echoes, which generally increases artifacts. (Feigenbaum-1)

2.2 T

2.3 T

2.4 F

2.5 T

Explanation for 2.2 through 2.5 Time-gain compensation is important in defining the septal border, the thickness of the right ventricular anterior wall, and right-sided valves. It allows the operator to adjust (compensate) for a stronger echo initially and weaker echoes farther into tissue. It does not selectively eliminate echoes (2.4) as the reject control does; instead it suppresses near-field stronger echoes and enhances far-field echoes, thereby compensating for attenuation of the ultrasound beam. (Feigenbaum-1)

2.6 T

2.7 F

2.8 T

2.9 F

Explanation for 2.6 through 2.9 Side lobes are a greater problem in phased-array systems because the number of small transducers used results in multiple edges. Each edge may generate radially directed sound energy, overlapping and producing artifacts. (Feigenbaum-1)

2.10 T

2.11 F

2.12 T

2.13 T

Explanation for 2.10 through 2.13 The only correct image in a parasternal long-axis plane is continuity between the interventricular septum and the anterior aortic root wall, as in 2.11. Answer 2.10 *might* be seen in an infarcted septum, and answer 2.12 *might* be seen in an intraventricular septal defect. However, when beginning an examination the sonographer should strive for aortoseptal continuity. Answer 2.13 is incorrect in all situations. (Feigenbaum-12)

2.14 B Contrast agents are more helpful in defining suspected shunts. (Feigenbaum-7)

2.15 F

2.16 T

2.17 F

2.18 T

Explanation for 2.15 through 2.18 It is true in answer 2.15 that contrast is totally filtered out at the pulmonary capillary level, but this does not affect the left-to-right shunt. Negative contrast, meaning an area of no contrast in the right chamber, is difficult to bring out in the echocardiogram. Some left-to-right shunts have a small right-to-left component that will show some contrast on the left side, but this is usually a small amount and not easy to define on the echocardiogram. (Weyman-12)

2.19 D Amyl nitrite may increase the systolic anterior motion (SAM) of the anterior mitral valve leaflet in IHSS. (See any general echocardiography text)

2.20 T

2.21 T

2.22 F

2.23 F

Explanation for 2.20 through 2.23 Neither inspiration nor expiration affects SAM, but both a Valsalva maneuver and amyl nitrite inhalation may bring it out. (Feigenbaum-9)

2.24 F

2.25 T

2.26 T

2.27 F

Explanation for 2.24 through 2.27 If the instrument allows changing the sample volume size, use a large sample volume for screening and a small sample volume for pinpointing the data. This often will shorten rather than lengthen the examination. (*Echocardiography* 1986; 3[6]:493)

2.28 C There is no single "easiest" location for Doppler imaging. The transducer is closer to the valves in the parasternal views. Since the Doppler beam is parallel to the mitral, aortic, and tricuspid valves at the apex, this is a good screening location. Since many jets are eccentric, it may not be true that "more" abnormalities are detected from the apex—a low parasternal view is used very successfully with color flow. (Nanda-6)

2.29 F Optimal Doppler angles are 0° or 180°. Parasternal views approximate angles of 90° giving a cosine ø (i.e., a multiplier) of 0.0. (Kisslo)

THREE

3.0 D All of the listed abnormalities can affect the size of the atrium. (See any general echocardiography text)

3.1 B In normal anatomy the mitral valve opens in diastole to a low-pressure left ventricle and fills rapidly. (Weyman-4)

3.2 F

3.3 F

3.4 T

3.5 T

Explanation for 3.2 through 3.5 The posterior leaflet of the mitral valve is smaller than the anterior leaflet and also scalloped. (Weyman-5)

3.6 F

3.7 F

3.8 T

3.9 T

Explanation for 3.6 through 3.9 Neither left atrial enlargement nor left atrial myxoma is indicated by the E–F slope. The pliability of the leaflets and free motion of the valve give an indication of any valvular stenosis. The rate of the slope will also be affected by changes in left ventricular function. (Feigenbaum-3)

3.10 F

3.11 T

3.12 T

3.13 F

Explanation for 3.10 through 3.13 Severe aortic insufficiency increases the left ventricular end-diastolic pressure, thereby diminishing the D–E point separation and highlighting the atrial component and the A kick. (Feigenbaum-6)

3.14 F Higher atrial pressures open the mitral valve. (Feigenbaum-4)

3.15 T

3.16 T

3.17 F

3.18 T

Explanation for 3.15 through 3.18 The mitral apparatus is composed of the mitral valve leaflets, chordae tendineae, papillary muscles, and mitral annulus. Fibrous bands can be found in the pericardial space of some patients with pericardial effusions. (Weyman-5)

3.19 C An increased A–C interval suggests increased left ventricular end-diastolic pressure (LVEDP) and possible poor left ventricular function. (Feigenbaum-4)

3.20 C With good imaging, measuring the mitral valve orifice in the parasternal short-axis plane provides reliable results. (Weyman-5)

3.21 T

3.22 T

3.23 F

3.24 F

Explanation for 3.21 through 3.24 The lateral and medial walls appear wider because of lateral resolution. Too high a gain setting will make the orifice too small. Transducer frequency and axial resolution do not affect the measurements. (Feigenbaum-6)

3.25 T

3.26 T

3.27 F

3.28 T

Explanation for 3.25 through 3.28 The color flow depiction of mitral stenosis shows a narrow jet with a blue central core (aliased) surrounded by yellow and red hues. It has been compared to a candle flame. (*Echocardiography* 1986; 3[6]:483)

3.29 B The apical four-chamber view allows the best angle for evaluating mitral valve flow. (Nanda-10)

3.30 C Left atrial enlargement is a direct physiological effect of mitral stenosis. (Feigenbaum-6)

3.31 D The surgeon distorts the valve at the time of commissurotomy, and the resultant morphology is not well visualized by two-dimensional echo. M mode has never been optimal for valve orifice determinations, and the Bernoulli equation gives velocity information but not orifice size. The most accurate way to determine valve size is with the pressure half-time equation. (Feigenbaum-6)

3.32 D All may cause improper closure of the valve. (Feigenbaum-6)

3.33 F

3.34 T

3.35 T

3.36 F

Explanation for 3.33 through 3.36 Flutter of the aortic leaflets in systole is frequently observed in normal subjects, so it is not considered to be abnormal motion. Early and also gradual systolic closure are frequently seen because of the reduced blood flow. (Feigenbaum-6)

3.37 T

3.38 T

3.39 F

3.40 T

Explanation for 3.37 through 3.40 Flutter of the interventricular septum is seen in aortic insufficiency, not mitral insufficiency. The rest are true: Left ventricular and left atrial enlargement and also flutter of the posterior aortic root may be observed. Pulsations of the right atrial wall may also be observed. (*Echocardiography* 1986; 3[2]:97)

3.41 B The peak mitral regurgitant velocity tells nothing about the degree of regurgitation, its etiology, or its direction—only the difference in pressure between the left ventricle and left atrium. (*Echocardiography* 1987; 4[4]:271)

3.42 B Mitral regurgitation causes a reduction in left ventricular outflow, thus reducing the amount of flow through the opening of the valve. The valve closes early. (Feigenbaum-6)

3.43 C Usually this is the better Doppler angle in relation to true flow. (Hatle-5)

3.44 T Left atrial enlargement is a direct physiological effect of mitral regurgitation. (Feigenbaum-6)

3.45 F Mitral regurgitation may be caused by a number of mitral valve problems. Mitral prolapse does not guarantee mitral regurgitation. (Feigenbaum-6)

3.46 D All could relate to poor valve closure. (Feigenbaum-6)

3.47 T

3.48 T

3.49 T

3.50 T

Explanation for 3.47 through 3.50 Each of the conditions described can be found in patients with papillary muscle dysfunction. The dilated mitral annulus may be the cause of the mitral regurgitation; the incomplete mitral closure is due to scarring of the papillary muscles secondary to myocardial infarction. And the papillary muscles shrink, pulling the chordae away from the mitral orifice. (Feigenbaum-6)

3.51 A The term *myxomatous degeneration* describes histologic changes seen in the mitral valve by the pathologist. The finding on echocardiography is thickening of the mitral leaflets. (Feigenbaum-6)

3.52 T

3.53 T

3.54 T

3.55 T

Explanation for 3.52 through 3.55 The listed findings can each be observed with flail mitral valve leaflets. (Feigenbaum-6)

3.56 T

3.57 T

3.58 F

3.59 T

Explanation for 3.56 through 3.59 The only described instance that does not produce doming is the flail mitral leaflet, which exhibits exaggerated, eccentric motion. (Weyman-5)

3.60 B The two-dimensional parasternal long-axis view displays the doming of the leaflets in mitral stenosis; the short-axis view may show normal separation of the leaflets. The E–F slope is not a sensitive predictor of mitral stenosis because it is also reduced in other conditions such as reduced left ventricular compliance. Lastly, although thickening of the mitral leaflets in the apical four-chamber view is seen on the mitral stenosis, the doming seen on parasternal long axis is a much better predictor of mitral stenosis. (Weyman-9)

3.61 F

3.62 T

3.63 T

3.64 F

Explanation for 3.61 through 3.64 Mitral annular calcification can obscure the posterior mitral valve leaflet because of the close proximity of these structures. Because of acoustic shadowing, the posterior left ventricular endocardium may also be obscured. (Feigenbaum-6)

3.65 T

3.66 T

3.67 T

3.68 T (Hatle-5)

3.69 B In mitral stenosis, early diastolic left ventricular filling is restricted, whereas the right ventricle fills rapidly. Therefore the septum bulges toward the left ventricle in early diastole. (Feigenbaum-6)

3.70 T

3.71 T

3.72 F

3.73 T

Explanation for 3.70 through 3.73 Patients with Marfan's syndrome exhibit a dilated aortic root with aortic regurgitation and mitral valve prolapse. Associated pulmonic regurgitation is not part of the syndrome. (*Echocardiography* 1986; 3[3]:255)

3.74 T

3.75 T

3.76 T

3.77 T

Explanation for 3.74 through 3.77 All of the choices influence mitral leaflet motion. (Weyman-5)

3.78 B The posterior leaflet usually moves anteriorly with the anterior leaflet, but if the leaflets are not fused, the posterior leaflet moves posteriorly. (Feigenbaum- 6)

3.79 T

3.80 T

3.81 T

3.82 F

Explanation for 3.79 through 3.82 Patients with aortic valve disease commonly exhibit a reduced E–F slope. This finding is believed to be related to a decreased rate of left ventricular filling associated with reduced left ventricular compliance. Mitral stenosis also exhibits a reduced E–F slope. In dilated cardiomyopathy, early closure of the mitral valve may be seen, but a reduced E–F slope is not. (Feigenbaum-6)

3.83 T

3.84 T

3.85 F

3.86 T

Explanation for 3.83 through 3.86 When imaging in the parasternal long-axis, the operator is prevented from adequately visualizing the valve orifice by doming of the anterior mitral leaflet. The parasternal short-axis is the proper position for measuring opening size. The operator must be careful with gain settings and ensure that the scan plane is parallel to and passes directly through the valve orifice. (*Echocardiography* 1986; 3[2]:109)

FOUR

4.0 T The left ventricle empties throughout systole, and the change in pressure with ventricular relaxation forces closure of the aortic valve. (Hagan-4)

4.1 A The aortic root undulates with the motion of the left ventricle. (See any general echocardiography text)

4.2 B The aortic valve leaflets are thickened. The left ventricular walls are hypertrophied, not normal thickness. The size of the left atrium is not affected by the aortic stenosis. The left ventricle has normal, not hypercontractile motion. (Weyman-7)

4.3 B The M mode cannot display doming, which can be seen only on the two-dimensional echocardiogram. The cusps frequently show normal separation and are not thickened or restricted. Diastolic separation of the cusps is seen in aortic regurgitation, not aortic stenosis. (Feigenbaum-6)

4.4 T

4.5 T

4.6 F

4.7 T

Explanation for 4.4 through 4.7 Shaggy echoes are noted with vegetations. Depending on the size and position of the jet(s) of aortic insufficiency, the mitral leaflet may flutter. If the volume of aortic insufficiency is such that the left ventricular pressure is increased, decreased separation of the mitral cusps as well as a decrease in the closing velocity can be seen. (See any general echocardiography text)

4.8 T

4.9 F

4.10 T

4.11 F

Explanation for 4.8 through 4.11 Rotating the patient does not necessarily help differentiate the source of the jets. Continuous-wave Doppler will show all signals simultaneously and will not distinguish the source. The intensity of the signal is less in aortic insufficiency than in mitral regurgitation; careful sampling in the left ventricular outflow tract and in the inflow tract should enable the operator to discern the correct source. (Kisslo-3)

4.12 C Aortic stenosis is defined by abnormal systolic echoes. (Feigenbaum-6)

4.13 B The parasternal short-axis view best defines the AV orifice, but the reliability of quantitation is debatable. (Feigenbaum-6)

4.14 C The suprasternal view provides the closest and most direct angle to AV outflow. (Levine et al.)

4.15 A The aortic flow velocity is increased with coexistent aortic insufficiency, which leads to overestimation of the gradient. (*Echocardiography* 1986; 3[1]: 3)

4.16 T

4.17 F

4.18 T

4.19 F

Explanation for 4.16 through 4.19 The formula $4 \times (V_2{}^2 - V_1{}^2)$ is important in calculating pressure drop when there is an increase in velocity in the left ventricular outflow tract and across the aortic valve, i.e., aortic stenosis and left ventricular outflow obstruction. (Hatle-5)

4.20 T

4.21 T

4.22 F

4.23 F

Explanation for 4.20 through 4.23 In patients with critical aortic stenosis but small gradients due to low stroke volume, the continuous-wave Doppler spectrum will demonstrate a later peak and symmetrical configuration. (*Echocardiography* 1986; 3[1]: 3)

4.24 T

4.25 F

4.26 T

4.27 T

Explanation for 4.24 through 4.27 All but aortic regurgitation will produce a high-velocity signal below the baseline when imaged from the apex. Aortic regurgitation will appear as a high-velocity signal above the baseline. (Hatle-5)

4.28 D Diastolic oscillations may not be associated with aortic stenosis. (Feigenbaum-6)

4.29 T (See any general cardiology text)

4.30 T Sclerotic valves tend to be dense but mobile. (Feigenbaum-6)

4.31 D Aortic regurgitant jets occur in the left ventricular outflow tract where the anterior leaflet of the mitral valve opens in diastole and the resultant flutter is noted on the M mode. (Feigenbaum-6)

4.32 D Left ventricular size may be expanded owing to the volume of aortic regurgitation. (Feigenbaum-6)

4.33 D This view is used because the angle of incidence is closest to 0° which gives the optimum Doppler angle and the greatest multiplier. (Hatle-5)

4.34 F This is *not* a finding associated with aortic regurgitation. (Feigenbaum-6)

4.35 T The bacterial infiltration may lead to poor closure of aortic cusps. (Weyman-7)

4.36 T

4.37 T

4.38 T

4.39 T

Explanation for 4.36 through 4.39 The sonographer should attempt all views, but usually the apical view is the least successful. (*Echocardiography* 1986; 3[6]: 483)

4.40 T

4.41 F

4.42 T

4.43 T

Explanation for 4.40 through 4.43 Underestimation occurs with reduced cardiac output when the maximum jet is not recorded and when the angle of incidence is increased. (Feigenbaum-4)

4.44 C The reason for early mitral valve closure in acute aortic insufficiency is elevated left ventricular diastolic pressure. Neither reduced cardiac output nor reduced left ventricular compliance affect mitral valve closure. The regurgitant jet of aortic insufficiency may affect mitral valve opening but will not cause early closure. (Feigenbaum-6)

4.45 F

4.46 T

4.47 T

4.48 T

Explanation for 4.45 through 4.48 Concentric left ventricular hypertrophy is related to aortic stenosis, not insufficiency. The effects of aortic regurgitation are increased septal motion, left ventricular dilatation, and sometimes septal flutter. (Feigenbaum-6)

4.49 F

4.50 T

4.51 T

4.52 F

Explanation for 4.49 through 4.52 Systolic flutter of the aortic leaflets is a normal finding. Flutter of the interventricular septum caused by aortic insufficiency is a diastolic, not a systolic, phenomenon. Diastolic leaflet flutter and diastolic left ventricular outflow tract echoes are seen with aortic insufficiency. (Feigenbaum-6)

4.53 C The term *reverse doming* refers to the convex curve sometimes observed on the two-dimensional echo of the mitral valve in the parasternal long-axis and/or apical view of patients with aortic regurgitation. (Feigenbaum-6)

4.54 T

4.55 F

4.56 T

4.57 T

Explanation for 4.54 through 4.57 Traditionally, aortic insufficiency is evaluated by the pulsed mapping technique. With insufficiency, the gradient does not help to determine the severity. A rapid pressure half-time means severe insufficiency. Last, color flow imaging of the thickness at the regurgitant stream at the valve is an accurate way of determining severity. (*Echocardiography* 1987; 4[4]: 271)

4.58 T

4.59 F

4.60 F

4.61 T

Explanation for 4.58 through 4.61 The Doppler aortic spectral waveform in *significant* aortic stenosis is late-peaking and symmetrical. If the aortic stenosis is less severe, the spectral waveform shows early peaking and a rapid descent, becoming asymmetrical. This is important in cases of combined aortic stenosis and insufficiency and also in cases of poor left ventricular function. (*Echocardiography* 1986; 3[1]: 3)

5.0 T Mitral valve dynamics usually occur prior to tricuspid valve dynamics. (Feigenbaum-7)

5.1 T

5.2 T

5.3 T

5.4 F

Explanation for 5.1 through 5.4 The M-mode criteria for tricuspid stenosis are similar to the pattern seen in mitral stenosis. (Feigenbaum-6)

5.5 T

5.6 T

5.7 T

5.8 T

Explanation for 5.5 through 5.8 See any general cardiology text.

5.9 C The suprasternal view may also be helpful, but the apical four-chamber view has a more accurate angle to flow. (Hatle-4)

5.10 C Right atrial enlargement is a direct physiological consequence of tricuspid stenosis. (Feigenbaum-6)

5.11 D None of the criteria are directly related. (Feigenbaum-6)

5.12 D Right atrial enlargement is a direct physiological consequence of tricuspid regurgitation, as it is of tricuspid stenosis. (Weyman-9)

5.13 C The apical four-chamber view gives the best angle for evaluating tricuspid regurgitation. (Feigenbaum-6)

5.14 B The tricuspid valve is the first valve contacted by returning blood flow to the heart and is therefore the valve where bacterial endocarditis most commonly occurs. (Feigenbaum-6)

5.15 T

5.16. F

5.17 T

5.18 F

Explanation for 5.15 through 5.18 The echo features of carcinoid heart disease in the tricuspid valve are thickened, rigid leaflets that do not close during systole, leaving wide-open tricuspid regurgitation. (Feigenbaum-6)

5.19 T

5.20 F

5.21 F

5.22 T

Explanation for 5.19 through 5.22 Scanning for the inferior vena cava and the hepatic vein is completed in the subcostal position. The presence of flow toward the transducer in systole when flow in the inferior vena cava and/or hepatic vein is being insonated is evidence for tricuspid regurgitation. Normal flow is always away from the transducer in diastole, with or without tricuspid regurgitation. (Feigenbaum-6)

5.23 B Contrast appears in the inferior vena cava on the M mode during ventricular systole with tricuspid regurgitation. It appears following atrial systole in normal subjects, and there is no contrast effect in diastole. (Feigenbaum-6)

5.24 F

5.25 T

5.26 T

5.27 F

Explanation for 5.24 through 5.27 Mitral valve inflow velocity in normal subjects is higher than tricuspid valve inflow velocity. Also, tricuspid inflow increases with inspiration. (Hatle-4)

5.28 F

5.29 T

5.30 T

5.31 F

Explanation for 5.28 through 5.31 Localized signals mean mild tricuspid regurgitation. Right atrial dimensions are increased in significant insufficiency. When the Doppler shows systolic flow into the hepatic veins, tricuspid regurgitation is significant. Tricuspid regurgitant jets frequently hug the interatrial septum, and this is not a sign of severity. (*Echocardiography* 1987; 4[4]: 271)

5.32 T

5.33 T

5.34 F

5.35 T

Explanation for 5.32 through 5.35 The velocity increases with inspiration in tricuspid stenosis. The other answers are all typical of tricuspid stenosis—increase in velocity that is mild compared with mitral stenosis; slow rate of descent of velocity curve following peak velocity; and diastolic dispersion. (Nanda-13)

5.36 B Right ventricular systolic pressure can be estimated by taking the peak velocity of the tricuspid regurgitant jet (in systole) and using the Bernoulli equation ($4V^2$) to predict peak right ventricular minus right atrial pressure gradients. By estimating mean right atrial pressure as 10 mmHg and adding that to the above findings, right ventricular systolic pressure is estimated. (Nanda-13)

5.37 B Tricuspid insufficiency will cause contrast to appear in the inferior vena cava and the hepatic veins during right ventricular systole. (Weyman-9)

5.38 F

5.39 T

5.40 T

5.41 F

Explanation for 5.38 through 5.41 The tricuspid valve opens before the mitral valve and closes after it. The earlier opening occurs because right ventricular pressure falls to the level of right atrial pressure sooner (peak systolic pressure is lower in the right ventricle than in the left). The tricuspid valve closes after the mitral valve because electrical activation of the left ventricle precedes that of the right ventricle. (Weyman-9)

5.42 B The three tricuspid valve leaflets are the anterior, the posterior, and the septal. In the parasternal right ventricular inflow view, the anterior and posterior are imaged. In the parasternal short-axis view, all three leaflets are imaged optimally. The apical four-chamber view demonstrates the anterior and septal leaflets. (Weyman-9)

5.43 T

5.44 F

5.45 T

5.46 F

Explanation for 5.43 through 5.46 The more apical insertion of the tricuspid septal leaflet relative to the mitral anterior leaflet distinguishes the right ventricle when there is any doubt. The tricuspid valve has three leaflets and also three papillary muscles, not four. (Weyman-9)

5.47 F

5.48 T

5.49 T

5.50 T

Explanation for 5.47 through 5.50 This group of acquired disorders presents on the echocardiogram with findings of tricuspid stenosis: thickened cordae, diastolic leaflet doming, and restriction of leaflet motion. The E:A ratio would be either decreased or, owing to lack of an A wave, nonexistent. (Weyman-9)

5.51 T

5.52 F

5.53 T

5.54 F

Explanation for 5.51 through 5.54 The parasternal long-axis right ventricular inflow view and the apical four-chamber view are the most reliable for viewing doming in tricuspid stenosis. The parasternal short-axis view is less reliable, although it may at times be domed. (Feigenbaum-6)

5.55 T

5.56 F

5.57 T

5.58 T

Explanation for 5.55 through 5.58 Dilatation of the right atrium occurs in tricuspid regurgitation but is not a sign of right ventricular volume overload. The other signs are all true of right ventricular volume overload. (Feigenbaum-6)

SIX

6.0 D Review cardiac anatomy in any general echocardiographic text.

6.1 C Other leaflets are usually not at the correct angle to the transducer. (Feigenbaum-2)

6.2 C The apical plane does not usually include the pulmonic valve. (See any general echocardiography text)

6.3 B The parasternal short-axis view usually offers the most appropriate angle to flow. (Hatle-5)

6.4 D See any general cardiology text.

6.5 T

6.6 T

6.7 F

6.8 T

Explanation for 6.6 through 6.8 The two-dimensional echo findings in pulmonic stenosis are the same as for other stenotic valves, i.e., doming leaflets, thickening of the structures, and leaflet tips that remain centrally positioned in systole. Eversion of the leaflets is seen in regurgitant lesions. (Feigenbaum-7)

6.9 F

6.10 T

6.11 T

6.12 T

Explanation for 6.9 through 6.12 The right ventricular outflow tract is described in terms of three levels: infundibular (subvalvular), valvular, and supravalvular. (Feigenbaum-7)

6.13 F

6.14 T

6.15 T

6.16 T

Explanation for 6.13 through 6.16 Disturbed flow would be proximal to the valve, not distal. The other answers are true signs of pulmonary hypertension: diffuse, disturbed signal proximal to the valve and an increased intensity of the continuous-wave Doppler waveform. (*Echocardiography* 1987; 4[4]: 271)

6.17 T

6.18 F

6.19 T

6.20 T

Explanation for 6.17 through 6.20 A pacemaker wire causes tricuspid regurgitation, not pulmonic regurgitation. The three other choices all cause pulmonary regurgitation. (Feigenbaum-7)

6.21 T

6.22 T

6.23 F

6.24 T

Explanation for 6.21 through 6.24 High-velocity disturbance of flow occurs in diastole, not systole. Also, acceleration time is shortened, so that the formula $80 - (AT \times .5)$ can be used to predict pulmonary hypertension. The decreased inflow in mid-systole corresponds to the notch seen on the M mode. (Feigenbaum-7)

6.25 A An exaggerated A wave, not absence of the A wave, is consistent with pulmonary stenosis. The absent A wave is consistent with pulmonary hypertension. Notching is also associated with pulmonary hypertension. Doming occurs on the two-dimensional examination, not on the M mode. (Feigenbaum-6)

6.26 D Normal pulmonary valve-flow velocity acceleration time is slower than aortic valve-flow velocity acceleration time. (Nanda-16)

6.27 T

6.28 T

6.29 T

6.30 F

Explanation for 6.27 through 6.30 Pulmonary regurgitation may cause a dilated right ventricle, but not dilatation of the right atrium. It also may cause flutter of the tricuspid leaflets just as aortic regurgitation may cause mitral valve flutter. Finally, the septal motion can become abnormal if right ventricular volume overload occurs. (Feigenbaum-6)

6.31 T

6.32 T

6.33 T

6.34 F

Explanation for 6.31 through 6.34 See any general echocardiography text.

7.0 T Echocardiography is a sensitive technique for identifying valvular vegetation. (Feigenbaum-6)

7.1 T

7.2 T

7.3 T

7.4 F

Explanation for 7.1 through 7.4 Vegetations have been observed echocardiographically in all of the listed instances except in the left atrial appendage. (Feigenbaum-6)

7.5 D A "trademark" of endocarditis is the normal motion of the valve leaflets. (Feigenbaum-6)

7.6 T

7.7 F

7.8 T

7.9 T

Explanation for 7.6 through 7.9 With mitral valve endocarditis one may see mitral valve prolapse, flail leaflets, and/or ruptured chordae tendineae. A left atrial thrombus, however, is not an associated finding; it is associated with mitral stenosis. (Weyman-5)

7.10 F

7.11 T

7.12 T

7.13 T

Explanation for 7.10 through 7.13 Intravenous drug abuse leads to endocarditis of the right sided valves, not the left. The common causes of aortic valve endocarditis include rheumatic deformity of the valve and calcification/degeneration of the aortic valves in the elderly. (Weyman-5)

7.14 F

7.15 T

7.16 T

7.17 T

Explanation for 7.14 through 7.17 No noninvasive method can determine the type of infection present in endocarditis. Two-dimensional echocardiography allows visualization of the size, shape, and exact location relative to other cardiac structures. (Weyman-5)

7.18 F

7.19 T

7.20 T

7.21 F

Explanation for 7.18 through 7.21 Mitral valve motion is preserved in endocarditis, and one sees an abnormal mass of echoes on the leaflets. Systolic leaflet separation is not a finding in endocarditis, only in some forms of mitral regurgitation (e.g., rheumatic). Eccentric motion from beat to beat is a feature of a flail mitral valve, not endocarditis. (Feigenbaum-6)

7.22 T

7.23 T

7.24 T

7.25 F

Explanation for 7.22 through 7.25 Vegetations from endocarditis on cardiac valves do not simply disappear, although they may embolize. They do erode and disrupt the valve and surrounding structures, and, if large enough, can obstruct valvular flow. (Weyman-5)

7.26 T

7.27 F

7.28 T

7.29 T

Explanation for 7.26 through 7.29 A myxoma is not a secondary finding of endocarditis. Fistulas, aneurysms, and abscesses may be secondary findings. (Feigenbaum-6)

7.30 F

7.31 T

7.32 T

7.33 F

Explanation for 7.30 through 7.33 The echocardiogram is helpful in visualizing the vegetations in endocarditis, but the lesions must be larger than 2 mm to be seen. Therefore the test is unable to detect abnormalities in the earliest stages. It is also unable to differentiate between old and new lesions. When a vegetation is observed, however, the sensitivity and specificity are quite high. (Feigenbaum-6)

EIGHT

8.0 C (Feigenbaum-6)

8.1 A M mode allows for direct measurement of prosthetic valve excursion. (Feigenbaum-6)

8.2 C The primary orifice is composed of the ring the ball sits in; the secondary orifice is between the ring and the ball; the tertiary orifice lies between the ball and the aortic wall. (Nanda-14)

8.3 T

8.4 T

8.5 F

8.6 T

Explanation for 8.3 through 8.6 The age of the valve is irrelevant to the Doppler hemodynamic evaluation of valvular stenosis. It is true that the bioprosthesis will stiffen with time, but when evaluating the prosthetic valve for degree of stenosis one considers the size of the valve and the patient for patient prosthesis mismatch as well as cardiac output—is it high or low? (Nanda-14)

8.7 F

8.8 T

8.9 T

8.10 F

Explanation for 8.7 through 8.10 Prosthetic valve motion is impeded when opening is incomplete or delayed. Swelling of old ball material restricts its motion, and thrombus formation also restricts motion. Deterioration of the valve material would cause erratic motion, not restriction. Dehiscence of a strut also causes erratic motion. (Feigenbaum-6)

8.11 F

8.12 T

8.13 T

8.14 T

Explanation for 8.11 through 8.14 All stenotic mitral valves demonstrate high peak velocity, slow decrease in diastolic velocity, and turbulent flow. A prosthetic valve that becomes stenotic functions the same. (Feigenbaum-6)

8.15 F

8.16 T

8.17 F

8.18 T

Explanation for 8.15 through 8.18 High prosthetic valve velocities are observed in high flow states such as increased cardiac output and valvular regurgitation. Congestive heart failure would cause reduced flow and increased left ventricular end-diastolic pressure but would not affect flow significantly. (Hatle-5)

8.19 F

8.20 T

8.21 T

8.22 T

Explanation for 8.19 through 8.22 There is no one correct position for recording the high velocity of the aortic prosthesis. One must make use of several approaches, that is, the apical, suprasternal, and right sternal border. Usually the left parasternal position is of no value in insonating flow in an aortic prosthesis. (Nanda-14)

8.23 F

8.24 T

8.25 T

8.26 F

Explanation for 8.23 through 8.26 The transprosthetic flow velocities are generally increased because prosthetic valves are all somewhat stenotic. To ensure recording of the true peak velocity and to avoid aliasing, it is best to record with the continuous-wave technique. Continuous-wave recordings do not localize a velocity. Note that ease of recording is not a valid reason for choosing a recording modality. (Nanda-14)

8.27 T

8.28 T

8.29 T

8.30 F

Explanation for 8.27 through 8.30 It is not abnormal to observe shadowing with any prosthetic valve apparatus. All other abnormalities noted can be observed with bioprostheses. (Weyman-5)

8.31 T

8.32 T

8.33 T

8.34 T

Explanation for 8.31 through 8.34 All of the listed configurations of prosthetic valves are currently in use. (Feigenbaum-6)

8.35 T

8.36 T

8.37 F

8.38 T

Explanation for 8.35 through 8.38 Thickening of bioprosthetic leaflets is not a normal observation; it has been observed in valvular stenosis, infectious endocarditis, and peripheral embolization. (Weyman-5)

8.39 B Only in the parasternal short-axis view can all three struts be seen. The struts are oriented 120° from each other, so in a plane that passes through the long-axis of the valve, only two struts can be seen. (Weyman-5)

8.40 B The term *dehiscence* refers to lack of attachment of a portion of the prosthetic valve to the heart. The condition produces a rocking, erratic motion on the echo. If valve leaflets appear in the left atrium in systole, the mitral prosthesis leaflet is flail. Thickened leaflets are associated with stenosis and endocarditis. The focal masses represent endocarditis. (Weyman-5)

8.41 C Rounding of the E point on the M mode of a Bjork-Shiley valve is abnormal and indicates some form of obstruction—either thrombosis or tissue ingrowth. It does not indicate regurgitation or a flail leaflet. A Bjork-Shiley valve is a tilting disk. (Feigenbaum-6)

9.0 C Constrictive pericarditis does not allow for flexible expansion of the left ventricle. (Feigenbaum-10)

9.1 F Although pericardial effusions can occur without posterior effusions, a good rule of thumb is to suspect pericardial effusion only when posterior effusions are noted as well. (Feigenbaum-10)

9.2 T

9.3 T

9.4 T

9.5 T

Explanation for 9.2 through 9.5 All of the above can be seen with tamponade. (Feigenbaum-10)

9.6 B An anterior echo-free space by itself does not identify pericardial effusion. (Feigenbaum-10)

9.7 T

9.8 T

9.9 T

9.10 T

Explanation for 9.7 through 9.10 All of the above. (Feigenbaum-10)

9.11 F

9.12 F

9.13 F

9.14 T

Explanation for 9.11 through 9.14 The density of echoes is too varied for either pericardial fat or an effusion. Also, the distance is not indicative of either entity. However, with an effusion the pericardium shows a flat pattern and does not remain a constant distance from the epicardium. (See any general echocardiography text)

TEN

10.0 C The myxoma may be tethered in such a way that it follows the flow from the left atrium into the left ventricle. The myxoma then appears as a structure posterior to the anterior mitral leaflet and, depending on its density, may be thought to be a thickening of the mitral leaflet. Two-dimensional echo helps to define the structures. (See any general echocardiography text)

10.1 D High-frequency oscillations are not noted in IHSS. (Feigenbaum-9)

10.2 C Dilated cardiomyopathy usually involves all myocardial cells. (Feigenbaum-9)

10.3 C To confirm a diagnosis of IHSS, both asymmetric septal hypertrophy (ASH) and systolic anterior motion (SAM) must be noted. (See any general echocardiography text)

10.4 B In right ventricular volume overload the septal motion becomes paradoxical. (See any general echocardiography text)

10.5 A "Beaking" is noted in left bundle branch block, Wolff-Parkinson-White syndrome, and right ventricular pacing. (Feigenbaum-5)

10.6 T

10.7 F

10.8 T

10.9 F

Explanation for 10.6 through 10.9 (See any general echocardiography text)

ELEVEN

11.0 F The role of echocardiography continues to increase in coronary artery disease, especially with the expanded role of stress echo. (Feigenbaum-8)

11.1 D In atrial fibrillation, each P wave generates an atrial contraction resulting in a constant reopening of the mitral valve that gives a sawtooth appearance. (See any general echocardiography text)

11.2 F

11.3 T

11.4 T

11.5 T

Explanation for 11.2 through 11.5 Right bundle branch block does not have the same effect on left ventricular conduction as left bundle branch block or Wolff-Parkinson-White syndrome. If electrical pacing is done in the right ventricular apex, beaking can be seen. (Feigenbaum-5)

11.6 B (See any general anatomy text)

11.7 F

11.8 T

11.9 F

11.10 T

11.11 T

Explanation for 11.7 through 11.11 Atherosclerosis is a generalized disease that begins most often at bifurcations because of the shear forces generated at the wall surfaces. Patients with atherosclerosis in the periphery will have other atherosclerotic changes in the carotid and coronary vessels even though these may be clinically silent. Of all the theories of its development, the injury/repair cycle seems to best account for the prevalence of coronary atherosclerotic disease found on postmortem examination of young men killed in Vietnam. Regardless of its etiology, there is no question that disruption of intimal continuity is the principal manifestation. (See any general anatomy text)

11.12 A (See any general anatomy text)

11.13 B Being female is not considered a risk factor although postmenopausal females are at greater risk for atherosclerosis than premenopausal females. (See any general cardiology text)

TWELVE

12.0 A The interatrial septum is best imaged in the subcostal long-axis plane, in which the beam is perpendicular to the septum. It also can be seen in the apical four-chamber and parasternal short-axis views. (Feigenbaum-7)

12.1 B The subcostal view provides a perpendicular angle from the transducer to the interatrial septum. This allows visualization of the primum, secundum, and fossa ovalis areas. The apical four-chamber view is parallel to the interatrial septum and often fails to record the area of the thin foramen ovalae because of "septal dropout." (Chang-7)

12.2 T Pressure is greater in the left atrium than in the right atrium, causing a slight bowing of the septum to the right. (Feigenbaum-3)

12.3 F As volume in the left atrium increases, the interatrial septum bows more toward the right atrial cavity. (Chang-7)

12.4 F In left atrial dilatation, the pressure is elevated in the left atrium, causing the interatrial septum to bulge toward the right atrium. (Levine et al.-13)

12.5 T Increased pressure in the right atrium will cause the interatrial septum to bow into the left atrial cavity. (Gardin & Talano-15)

12.6 B The most common congenital cardiac lesion that can be documented by echocardiography in early adulthood is an atrial septal defect. (Feigenbaum-7)

12.7 C The thin part of the interatrial septum, the ostium secundum area, is the most common site of atrial septal defects. The other sites are the primum septum and the sinus venous area. (Hagan-8)

12.8 C The most common atrial septal defect shows a left-to-right shunt, an enlarged right atrium and ventricle, a flat or paradoxical interventricular septal motion, and broadening at the edges of the septal defect. (Levine et al.-13)

12.9 F The apical four-chamber view is the more useful in evaluating the primum septum and membranous septum. (Feigenbaum-3)

12.10 T Muscular defects may be difficult to visualize, as they tend to be very small. However, if the defect is 2 mm or more, the apical four-chamber or subcostal long-axis planes may be the best for imaging of the muscular septum. (Hagan-9)

12.11 F The septal thickness should be compared to the posterior wall thickness in the parasternal long- or short-axis views because the transducer beam is more perpendicular to the myocardial tissue in these views. (Feigenbaum-3)

12.12 F There are several windows useful for visualizing an aneurysm in the membranous septal area. The parasternal long-axis and apical four-chamber views are very useful. The short-axis view may image the aneurysm, but less easily than the other views. (Feigenbaum-3)

12.13 C Ventricular septal defects are the most common congenital malformation of the heart. They may be small (located in the muscular septum) and may close spontaneously with age. (Hagan-9)

12.14 T Membranous ventricular septal defects are divided at this anatomic plane and may be classified as subaortic or subpulmonic. (Hagan-9)

12.15 T Supracristal defects lie immediately below the aortic valve, with the valve forming the superior margin of the defect. (Hagan-9)

12.16 T Small muscular defects are very common, with spontaneous closure occurring with time. (Hagan-9)

12.17 F Membranous defects may arise only in the area of the thin membranous septum. They may be small or large, single or multiple. (Kisslo-12)

12.18 F Multiple small defects can cause a clinically significant volume overload on the heart. (Hagan-9)

12.19 F Overriding of the aortic root usually occurs when the aorta is dilated (as in tetralogy of Fallot or truncus arteriosus). A membranous septal defect may be present with these conditions, but a defect may occur without aortic root dilatation and override. (Feigenbaum-7)

12.20 A The endocardial cushions play a significant role in the embryologic development of the septum primum, atrioventricular valves, and membranous septum. (Kisslo-13)

12.21 E Prolapse of the aortic valve is visualized in the presence of a sinus of Valsalva aneurysm, a high perimembranous ventricular septal defect, or a supracristal ventricular septal defect. (Levine et al.-13)

12.22 A Hypoplasia of the ascending aorta causes localized or diffuse narrowing of the vessel distal to the coronary arteries. (Gardin & Talano-16)

12.23 C A patent ductus arteriosus will produce a high-pitched positive Doppler flow in diastole if the shunt is left to right. (Feigenbaum-7)

12.24 B There are four common findings in a patient with tetralogy of Fallot. The degree of pulmonic stenosis may vary from mild to severe (cyanotic). (Feigenbaum-7)

12.25 C A discrete subaortic membrane may be best seen on the parasternal long-axis or four-chamber view. It may be complete or partial. The amount of obstruction will determine the degree of left ventricular pressure. (Chang-7)

12.26 D Most aortic coarctations occur at the level of the left subclavian artery. (Feigenbaum-7)

12.27 B Transposition of the great arteries occurs when there is a malrotation of the great vessels and the pulmonary artery arises from the left ventricle while the aorta arises from the right ventricle. (Hagan-13)

12.28 C Ebstein's anomaly is characterized by a huge right atrial cavity secondary to an incompetent tricuspid valve. The apically displaced tricuspid valve is separated from the atrial cavity by an "atrialized" chamber of the right ventricle. (Weyman-9)

12.29 D Pulmonic stenosis is characterized by thickened, domed leaflets. The M-mode tracing shows a prominent "a" dip (more than 7 mm). The Doppler tracing is very harsh, over 2 m/s. (Clark-5)

12.30 B The failure of the right ventricular outflow tract to develop completely results in pulmonary atresia. It is usually associated with right ventricular and tricuspid valvular hypoplasia, with a right-to-left shunt at the atrial level. (Hagan-3)

12.31 D In tricuspid atresia, the left ventricle is enlarged, and all systemic venous return is shunted right to left at the atrial level, usually through a large patent foramen ovale or an atrial septal defect. (Hagan-3)

12.32 E The atrial septal defect will cause a volume overload on the right heart (with a left-to-right shunt). This causes the septal motion to be abnormal. (Gardin & Talano-15)

12.33 D The dilated structure posterior to the left atrial cavity is the coronary sinus. This structure is dilated in patients with a persistent left superior vena cava, as this structure drains into the coronary sinus. (Feigenbaum-3)

12.34 B In cor triatriatum, a subdivision exists within the left atrial cavity, obstructing pulmonary venous return; however, the pulmonary veins do enter the left atrial cavity. (Hagan-4)

12.35 A A defect in the endocardial cushion area may be indicated by absence of the primum septum or the membranous septum. The atrioventricular valves may be malformed with resultant regurgitation. (Levine et al.-13)

12.36 C The presence of a ventricular septal defect may cause abnormal development of the chordal attachments of the atrioventricular valve. The straddling atrioventricular valve means the chordal attachment crosses the ventricular septal defect into the opposite ventricular cavity. (Hagan-9)

12.37 D Aortic atresia is hypoplasia (underdevelopment) of the left ventricle. This causes the aortic root to be very small with severe aortic obstruction. (Feigenbaum-7)

12.38 C Hypertrophied muscle bands within the right ventricular outflow tract would cause obstruction through the pulmonary artery, and thus an increased Doppler velocity tracing would be obtained. (Clark-5)

12.39 D Parachute mitral valve is a form of infravalvular obstruction in which the papillary muscles are closer than normal or fused to form a single papillary muscle. The chordae tendineae are usually thickened, short, and fused, causing further obstruction. The lesion is usually associated with congenital mitral stenosis. (Kisslo-17)

THIRTEEN

13.0 C Frequency is a source-dependent phenomenon. (Kremkau-2)

13.1 T

13.2 T

13.3 F

13.4 F

13.5 T

Explanation for 13.1 through 13.5 Sound is described by the parameters of frequency, period, wavelength, propagation speed, amplitude, and intensity. (Kremkau-2)

13.6 A Batteries deliver direct current unless the voltage is put through an alternator. Household current alternates at 60 hertz. (See any general physics text)

13.7 B (Kremkau-2)

13.8 D (Kremkau-2)

13.9 A (Kremkau-2)

13.10 A (Kremkau-2)

13.11 D (Kremkau-2)

13.12 C Frequency is the number of times a complete cycle passes a point of reference, hence 5 hertz (Hz), which is equal to 5 cycles per second (c/s). (Kremkau-2)

13.13 D Period is the reciprocal of frequency, or 1 divided by the frequency. (Kremkau-2)

13.14 A (Kremkau-3)

13.15 B (Kremkau-2, or see any ultrasound text)

13.16 T

13.17 T

13.18 F

13.19 T

Explanation for 13.16 through 13.19 Frequency is defined as the number of regular recurrences in a given time such as the frequency of the heartbeat. In describing sound, frequency is notated in hertz: One (1) hertz, or 1 Hz, is equal to 1 cycle per second; 1 kilohertz, (kHz) is equal to 1000 c/s; 1 megahertz, or 1 MHz, is equal to 1 million hertz or 1 million c/s. (See any general physics text)

13.20 C (Kremkau-2)

13.21 D (Kremkau-2)

13.22 A Watts per square centimeter (W/cm^2) is the terminology for describing acoustic power output such as the Doppler-probe output. Safe upper limits for Doppler probes are 100 milliwatts per square centimeter of tissue (100 mW/cm^2). (Kremkau-5)

13.23 C (Kremkau-2)

13.24 B Another way of looking at this equation is:

$$I = 4/2 \quad or \quad 2.$$

(Kremkau-Appendix D)

13.25 D Another way of looking at this equation is:

$$E = I \times R \quad or \quad E = 36.$$

(Kremkau-Appendix D)

13.26 C Another way of of looking at this question is:

$$R = I/E \quad or \quad 56/28 \quad or \quad R = 2.$$

(Kremkau-Appendix D)

13.27 B Let's look at the answer to this question by solving it. Assume that the following equation is the baseline:

$$80 = 100 - (10 \times 2) \quad \text{or} \quad 80 = 100 - 20.$$

If we double Q to 20 the equation will read

$$60 = 100 - (20 \times 2)$$

Because of the minus sign in front of the $Q \times R_{seg}$ section this has an inverse function on P_2. Therefore when Q or R_{seg} increases, P_2 decreases. Conversely, when Q or R_{seg} decreases, P_2 increases.

13.28 D

13.29 A

13.30 D

13.31 B

13.32 C Since the radius is to the fourth power, if the radius is decreased by 50% the resistance increases to the fourth power, or 16 times. A way of illustrating this is as follows:

$$4 \times 4 \times 4 \times 4 = 256, \ 2 \times 2 \times 2 \times 2 = 16, \ 16 \times 16 = 256$$

13.33 E (See any general physics text)

13.34 A A Doppler beam at 90° to blood flow does not produce a frequency shift because the cosine of the angle is zero, and therefore the multiplier within the Doppler equation is zero. Because of random motion, however, this physical fact may not translate into a situation of no flow while the Doppler beam is at 90° to the flow. (Kremkau-Appendix C)

FOURTEEN

14.0 E The propagation speed most used in cardiac technology is the propagation speed of sound in soft tissue, 1540 meters per second (m/s). (Kremkau-2)

14.1 B (Kremkau-2)

14.2 C (Kremkau-2)

14.3 B (Kremkau-2)

14.4 B (Kremkau-2)

14.5 C The constant used in solving the Doppler equation is 1540 m/s. (See any general ultrasound text)

14.6 D The liver, fat, muscle, and subcutaneous tissue are all soft tissues. In soft tissue the propagation speed of sound is averaged at 1540 m/s. (Feigenbaum-1 or general ultrasound text)

14.7 B Attenuation is the reduction of the strength of any sound beam. Your voice is more attenuated when it reaches someone across the room than when it reaches someone next to you. (Feigenbaum-1 or any physics text)

14.8 A Attenuation is a function of reflection and scattering of sound waves as well as changes in tissue characteristics (interfaces). Depth of ultrasound penetration affects the attenuation at no less than 1/dB/cm/MHz. (Feigenbaum-1)

14.9 C (See any general ultrasound text)

14.10 D Attenuation is defined by absorption, scattering, and reflection. (Kremkau-2 or any ultrasound text)

14.11 B A greater rate of signal attenuation occurs with higher-frequency transducers. (See any general ultrasound text)

14.12 B (Feigenbaum-1)

14.13 D Cathode ray (CRT) monitors can display only a fixed quantity of information at a single time; at present this level is established at approximately 36 dB. (Feigenbaum-1)

FIFTEEN

15.0 A (Kremkau-2)

15.1 E (Kremkau-2)

15.2 B (Kremkau-Appendix B)

15.3 D (Kremkau-Appendix B)

15.4 A (Feigenbaum-1)

15.5 C (Kremkau-4)

15.6 E (Feigenbaum-1)

15.7 E (Feigenbaum-1 or any ultrasound text)

15.8 A Zone of sensitivity is the term used for continuous-wave (CW) Doppler. Sample volume is the term used with pulsed Doppler systems. (See any general ultrasound text)

15.9 E The frequency of a crystal is determined by its size and shape. Piezoelectric crystals are stimulated electronically by an oscillator of a known frequency to induce the resonant frequency of the crystal. (Feigenbaum-1)

15.10 B The principles here are the same as with any light source. If you focus any light source with its power remaining static, the intensity increases at the point of focus. (Kremkau-2)

15.11 D Mechanical and array-type systems are differentiated by the means used to arc the beam through tissue. (Feigenbaum-1)

15.12 F

15.13 T

15.14 T

15.15 F

Explanation for 15.12 through 15.15 Axial resolution is the determinate that improves acuity in separating structures side by side along the propagation axis of the ultrasound beam. (Feigenbaum-1)

15.16 C Shorter bursts of ultrasound are less likely to overlap upon subsequent reflection from closely spaced structures than are longer bursts. (Feigenbaum-1)

15.17 T

15.18 T

15.19 F

15.20 F

15.21 F

Explanation for 15.17 through 15.21 Lateral resolution is purely a function of ultrasound beam width, a product of transmission frequency selected and the system's acoustical gathering capacity (a function of focal length and transducer diameter). (Feigenbaum-1)

15.22 C Only two axes exist in a given two-dimensional plane: X and Y. Clinically, these terms are translated into axial and lateral. (Feigenbaum-1)

SIXTEEN

16.0 C M-mode echo display offers the observer opportunity to study the patterns of motion produced by dynamic structures. No reliable morphologic data are provided. (Feigenbaum-1)

16.1 T

16.2 F

16.3 F

16.4 F

Explanation for 16.1 through 16.4 An A-mode echo display simplifies information from reflective targets along a single beam vector. (Feigenbaum-1)

16.5 C (Feigenbaum-1)

16.6 C (Feigenbaum-1)

16.7 C (Feigenbaum-1)

16.8 C B-mode real-time instrumentation is a product of the electronic evolution of noninvasive technology, providing rapidly updated images of tissue. (Feigenbaum-1)

16.9 D B-mode imaging is a two-dimensional modality that additionally provides signal amplitude data. (Feigenbaum-1)

16.10 T

16.11 F

16.12 F

16.13 T

Explanation for 16.10 through 16.13 The separate electronic requirements of computer processing and CRT monitor display require that both analog and digital scan-conversion circuitry be used within most current systems. (Kremkau-5)

16.14 T

16.15 F

16.16 T

16.17 F

Explanation for 16.14 through 16.17 Digital scan conversion is simply a process of making the input electronic signal from the imaging probe computer-ready, allowing virtually unlimited mathematical processing of the digitized signal. (Kremkau-5)

16.18 B An analog scan conversion system allows for "fluid" compression of the input image signal, smoothing the apparent differences in the subsequently displayed image. (Kremkau-5)

17.0 C (Kremkau-2)

17.1 B (Kremkau-2)

17.2 B High-frequency Dopplers have more attenuation owing to the stated equation. For a 20 MHz Doppler ultrasound device, the minimum attenuation would be 20 dB/cm. (Kremkau-2)

17.3 D Refer to the Doppler-shift formula. (Kremkau-2)

17.4 C Although analog strip chart recorders give the appearance of limited Doppler frequencies, evidence of the numerous frequencies obtainable from the Doppler signal is seen while using spectrum analysis. (Kremkau-2)

17.5 A (Kremkau-1 or any ultrasound text)

17.6 E The reflected frequency might be one-half the incident frequency (depending on the speed of the reflector), but it would always be less than the incident frequency. (Kremkau-7)

17.7 C A 0° angle causes the greatest Doppler shift owing to the function of the angle of incidence (cosine theta). Theoretically, a 90° angle of incidence will produce no reflected Doppler signal. In cardiac applications, the optimum Doppler angle of 0° is used to evaluate blood flow. (Kremkau-2)

17.8 B To state it in another way, antegrade flow is flow toward the Doppler probe tip and retrograde flow is flow away from the Doppler probe tip. (Kremkau-2)

17.9 A The angle of incidence is the single most difficult factor to determine while using Doppler ultrasound for regular noninvasive testing, mainly because the course of the blood vessel under the skin is unknown. This limitation does not apply to modern duplex scanning techniques, since a precise angle of incidence may be obtained. (Kremkau-2)

17.10 B The pulse repetition frequency (PRF) of a pulsed Doppler system limits the maximum detectable Doppler frequency to PRF/2. This means that a PRF of 11 kHz will alias (fold over) all Doppler frequencies over 5.5 kHz. With a shifted Doppler frequency of 6 kHz and a PRF of 11 kHz the frequencies between 5.5 and 6 kHz will be "folded." (Feigenbaum-1)

17.11 B Although the frequency received is affected by the angle of incidence (cosine theta) and the speed of sound in tissue, the answer to this question is received frequency. (Feigenbaum-1 or any ultrasound text)

17.12 A The continuous-wave (CW) Doppler may be used to determine blood flow if the arterial diameter is a known quantity. All Dopplers can detect a frequency shift and all directional Dopplers determine the direction of velocity changes. Spectral analysis is only a display mode and functions regardless of the type of Doppler being used. Only the pulsed Doppler with its gated, timed pulses of ultrasound can be used for depth location. (Feigenbaum-1 or any ultrasound text)

17.13 C It is important to remember that the spectrum analyzer is a method of display and that although it can detect velocity shifts caused by two or more vessels, background noise, and arterial wall motion, it is unable to indicate whether a vessel is being fully insonated. (Hatle-3)

17.14 T (Kremkau-7)

17.15 T (Kremkau-7)

17.16 F Acoustic interfaces may affect the attenuation of the signal but do not determine the sample size. (Kremkau-7)

17.17 T (Kremkau-7)

17.18 F The analog outputs affect only the manner in which information is processed once received. (Kremkau-7)

17.19 C The term *zero crossing* refers to a method of discriminating between antegrade and retrograde velocity information from which the mean frequency is determined. *Bidirectional* and *unidirectional* describe the ability of a Doppler device to detect antegrade and retrograde shifts (only the bidirectional Doppler detects both). *Fast Fourier transform* is a method of analyzing the separated Doppler signal. (Feigenbaum-1)

17.20 C (Hatle-3)

17.21 E Capacitance is not a term used to describe the output from a Doppler ultrasound device. (Hatle-3)

17.22 B (Hatle-3)

17.23 E Doppler signals are converted into analog signals by zero-crossing detectors or quadrature-phase detectors. Fast Fourier transform is a mathematical method of analyzing Doppler data and preparing velocity distributions for display. (Hatle-3)

17.24 B The flow-velocity profile contains many velocity elements at varying frequencies. The separation of these individual elements yields more statistical data than does the "averaging" process of the zero crossing detector's root mean square output. (Hatle-3)

17.25 A Fast Fourier transform spectral analysis is a statistical extrapolation process that operates independently of direction of blood flow or equipment used to input into the equation. (Hatle-3)

17.26 T

17.27 F

17.28 T

17.29 F

Explanation for 17.26 through 17.29 The sum total energy output from a system in intermittent operation is inherently less than a system that operates continuously. Ultrasound cannot penetrate the big bony structures of the cervical spine. Flow velocity analysis is accomplished by completion of information in the algebraic Doppler velocity equation and is unrelated to the specific instrumentation used. (See any general ultrasound text)

17.30 T Depth differentiation can be done only with pulsed Doppler. (Kremkau-7)

17.31 T (Kremkau-7)

17.32 T One way to look at a Doppler transducer and determine whether it is continuous-wave or pulsed is by observing the number of transducers on its face.

17.33. F Aliasing occurs only in pulsed Doppler systems. (Kremkau-7)

17.34 C (Kremkau-7)

17.35 D Any movement between the transmission source and target site will produce a Doppler frequency shift. (Kremkau-7)

17.36 T The transmitted frequency. (Kremkau-7)

17.37 T Or cosine theta. (Kremkau-7)

17.38 F Flow direction is not a variable in the Doppler flow velocity equation. (Kremkau-7)

17.39 T (Kremkau-7)

17.40 B (Hatle-3)

17.41 B Aliasing occurs as a "fold over" of Doppler signals and takes place above one-half the pulse repetition frequency or PRF/2. (Hatle-3)

17.42 A Only continuous-wave Doppler systems, regardless of additional instrumentation used, can faithfully recreate the instantaneous changes that occur in the blood flow velocity profile. (Hatle-3)

17.43 D (Hatle-3)

17.44 C This value is also referred to as the Nyquist limit. (Hatle-3)

17.45 B (Hatle-3)

17.46 F

17.47 F

17.48 T

17.49 T

Explanation for 17.46 through 17.49 Aliasing occurs at *all* frequencies above PRF/2 (the Nyquist limit) which in this case equals 7.5 kHz. (Hatle-3)

17.50 F

17.51 T

17.52 T In order to get a falsely low peak frequency.

17.53 F

Explanation for 17.50 through 17.53 Operator-induced minimization of the maximum frequency shift may reduce it to a level below the Nyquist limit (PRF/2). (Kremkau-8)

17.54 D (Hatle-3)

17.55 D (Kremkau-7)

17.56 C Since continuous-wave Dopplers insonate the entire vessel, one would expect reduced windowing when the signal is used in spectral analysis. Continuous-wave Dopplers obtain velocity information from throughout the insonated section, and since there can be many different velocities within this section this may cause decreased windowing when compared with a pulsed Doppler system that is insonating only a discrete section of velocities. (Kremkau-7)

17.57 D The Doppler formula includes all of the listed variables except blood flow. (See any general ultrasound text)

17.58 C In a time-domain spectrum analyzer, each frequency is represented on the screen. With a constant pure tone, each will appear as a straight line. (Hatle-3)

17.59 A It is important to remember to keep both delta F and F consistent in units so that if delta F is given as 4.6 kHz, then 2 MHz becomes 2000 kHz. In addition, if $\phi = 45$ then $\cos \phi = 0.70$ and the equation is:

$4.6 \times 1540 \ / \ (2 \times 2000 \times 0.70)$
or
$7084/2800$ which is 2.53 m/s

(Nanda-Appendix 11)

17.60 D The equation is:

$6.8 \times 1540/(2 \times 3000 \times 0.70)$
or
$10472/4200 = 2.49$ m/s

(Nanda-Appendix 11)

17.61 E The equation is:

$12.2 \times 1540/(2 \times 2500 \times 0.70)$
or
$18788/3500 = 5.36$ m/s

(Nanda-Appendix 11)

17.62 B Remember that cosine ø of 0° is 90. The equation is:

$4.6 \times 1540/2 \times 3000 \times 0.90$
or
$7084/5400 = 1.31$ mm/s

(Nanda-Appendix 11)

17.63 A The equation for velocity is:

$6.7 \times 1540 / (2 \times 3000 \times 0.90)$
or
$10318/5400$
or
1.91 m/s

This gives $4 \times (1.91)^2$ to find the pressure gradient of 14.59.

$4 \times (1.91 \times 1.91)$
or
$4 \times 3.65 = 14.60$

(Nanda-Appendix 11)

17.64 E Equation is:

$10 \times 1540/(2 \times 2000 \times 0.70)$
or
$15400/2800 = 5.5$ m/s

$P_1 - P_2 = 4 \times (5.5)^2$
or
pressure gradient $= 4 \times (5.5 \times 5.5) = 4 \times 30.25 = 121$ mmHg

(Nanda-Appendix 11)

EIGHTEEN

18.0 A (Kremkau-3)

18.1 D The magnitude of acoustical mismatch between the vessel wall and liquid blood is the same; it is independent of the order in which the ultrasound beam strikes them. (Kremkau-8)

18.2 D Sound is transmitted through the body according to the ability of tissues to transmit vibratory energy. Bony structures are highly resistant to this vibratory process because of their rigid composition. (Kremkau-8)

18.3 D The reflection coefficient of red blood cells is extremely poor. With an angle of zero and a blood velocity of 15.4 cm/s, a 5 MHz Doppler ultrasound signal will be shifted only 1000 Hz. That is, only 1000 Hz will be received from the 5 million Hz transmitted. (Kremkau-3)

NINETEEN

19.0 T

19.1 T

19.2 F

19.3 T

19.4 T

Explanation for 19.0 through 19.4 Acoustic output is necessary when considering bioeffects and safety, not for performance measurements. (Kremkau-9)

19.5 C Relative system sensitivity is discovered by finding the lowest gain or attenuation setting with no compensation at which a particular rod in the AIUM phantom produces a barely decernible display. (Kremkau-9)

19.6 F

19.7 T

19.8 F

19.9 T

19.10 F

Explanation for 19.6 through 19.10 Axial resolution from the AIUM test object is done from face A on pod group (a) with separations of from 1 mm to 5 mm. The resolution thus obtained is usually not reflective of the best possible resolution of the instrument. (Kremkau-9)

19.11 A When the AIUM test object is used, any rod may be employed to measure gray-scale dynamic range. (Kremkau-9)

19.12 E Heat results from thermal molecular motion, is equal to intensity multiplied by time, and is expressed in joules/cm². (Kremkau-Appendix D)

19.13 C Frequency is determined by the propagation speed of the transducer material and the thickness of the transducer element. (Kremkau-4)

TWENTY

20.0 C (Kremkau-10)

20.1 A Molecules moving back and forth along their axis do create heat. There is no disruption of cell walls at ultrasound frequencies below 100 mW/cm². (Kremkau-10)

20.2 B The product of intensity multiplied by time is expressed in heat or joules. The correct answer is less than 50 joules/cm². (Kremkau-10)

BIBLIOGRAPHY

TWO-DIMENSIONAL AND M-MODE

Chang S. *Echocardiography: Techniques and Interpretation,* 2nd ed. Philadelphia: Lea & Febiger, 1981.

Chung EK. *Quick Reference to Cardiovascular Diseases,* 2nd ed. Philadelphia: JB Lippincott, 1987.

Clark R. *Case Studies in Echocardiography.* Philadelphia: WB Saunders, 1977.

Feigenbaum H. *Echocardiography,* 4th ed. Philadelphia: Lea & Febiger, 1986.

Gardin J, Talano J. *Textbook of Two-Dimensional Echocardiography.* Orlando, FL: Grune & Stratton, 1983.

Hagan AD, DiSessa TG, Bloor CM, et al. *Two-Dimensional Echocardiography: Clinical and Pathological Correlations in Adolescent and Adult Heart Disease.* Boston: Little, Brown, 1983.

Weyman A. *Cross Sectional Echocardiography.* Philadelphia: Lea & Febiger, 1982.

DOPPLER

Hatle L, Angelsen B. *Doppler Ultrasound in Cardiology: Physical Principles and Clinical Applications,* 2nd ed. Philadelphia: Lea & Febiger, 1985.

Kisslo J, Adams D, Belkin R. *Doppler Color Flow Imaging.* New York: Churchill Livingstone, 1988.

Kisslo J, Adams D, Marks D. *Basic Doppler Echocardiography.* London: Churchill Livingstone, 1986.

Labovitz A, Williams G. *Doppler Echocardiography, Quantitative Methods of Pulsed and Continuous Wave Cardiac Doppler,* 2nd ed. Philadelphia: Lea & Febiger, 1988.

Levine R, Parlman A, Brown S, Jenko C. *Two-Dimensional Doppler Echocardiographic Technique.* Los Angeles: Great American Printing, 1984.

Nanda N. *Doppler Echocardiography: The Book.* New York: Igaku-Shoin, 1985.

Omoto R. *Color Atlas of Real-Time and Two-Dimensional Doppler Echocardiography,* 2nd ed. Philadelphia: Lea & Febiger, 1984.

PHYSICS OF DOPPLER IMAGING

Kremkau F. *Diagnostic Ultrasound: Principles, Instrumentation, and Exercises,* 2nd ed. Orlando, FL: Grune & Stratton, 1984.

ADDITIONAL REFERENCES

Allen HD, Marx GR. Doppler Echocardiography in Pediatric Cardiology. In Kisslo J, Adams D, Belkin R (eds), *Doppler Color Flow Imaging.* New York: Churchill Livingstone, 1988.

Hagen-Ansert SL. *Textbook of Diagnostic Ultrasonography,* 3rd ed. St. Louis: CV Mosby, 1988.

McDicken W. *Diagnostic Ultrasonics: Principles and Use of Instruments.* New York: John Wiley & Sons, 1981.

Reneman RS, Hoeks APG. *Doppler Ultrasound in the Diagnosis of Cerebrovascular Disease.* Chichester, England: Research Studies Press, 1982.

Sahn DJ, Anderson F. *Two-Dimensional Anatomy of the Heart.* New York: John Wiley & Sons, 1982.

Wicks JD, Howe KS. *Fundamentals of Ultrasonographic Techniques.* Chicago: Year Book Medical Publishers, 1983.

Williams RG, Tucker CR. *Echocardiographic Diagnosis of Congenital Heart Disease.* Boston: Little, Brown, 1977.